DISABLING LAWS, ENABLING ACTS
Disability Rights in Britain and America

CAROLINE GOODING

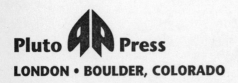

Pluto Press
LONDON • BOULDER, COLORADO

First published 1994 by Pluto Press
345 Archway Road, London N6 5AA
and 5500 Central Avenue
Boulder, Colorado 80301, USA

British Library Cataloguing in Publication Data
A Catalogue record for this book is available from the British Library

ISBN 0 7453 0770 1 hardback

Law and Social Theory
ISSN 1351-5020

Library of Congress Cataloging in Publication Data
Gooding, Caroline, 1959–
      Disability, discrimination and the law / Caroline Gooding.
        p.   cm. — (Law and social theory, ISSN 1351–5020)
      Includes bibliographical references and index.
      ISBN 0–7453–0770–1 (hardback)
      1. Discrimination against the handicapped—Law and legislation
—Great Britain. 2. Handicapped—Legal status, laws, etc.—Great
Britain. 3. Discrimination against the handicapped—Law and
legislation—United States. 4. Handicapped—Legal status, laws,
etc.—United States.   I. Title. II. Series.
      KD737.G57   1994
      342.73'087—dc20
      [347.30287]   94–26208
                                                             CIP

98 97 96 95 94
 6   5   4   3   2   1

Designed and Produced for Pluto Press by
Chase Production Services, Chipping Norton, OX7 5QR
Typeset from author's disks by
Stanford Desktop Publishing Services, Milton Keynes
Printed in Finland by WSOY

Disabling Laws, Enabling Acts

Law and Social Theory
A Pluto series

Series editor PETER FITZPATRICK
Professor of Law and Social Theory, University of Kent

Contents

To Mandy and Heidi who were there at the book's conception, and to Anne for assisting with its protracted birth

Acknowledgements

This book is based on an LLM Thesis which I wrote while at the University of California at Berkeley, 1990–1. My thanks are due to the American Association of University Women and the Fulbright Commission for funding my studies, to Riva Siegel for supervising them, and to Mme Christopher and Commander Hirschkron for making my stay so memorable.

I am grateful to Professor Peter Fitzpatrick for commissioning this book, and for his ongoing support and enthusiasm, and to Alastair McQueen and Jonathan Harris for their encouragement and advice, without which I might have given up looking. Further thanks are due to Barry for technical support, and Clare Goodridge and Paul Simpson for their comments on the housing and education sections.

Ultimately, this book stems from the disability movement. To anyone familiar with their work, my debt to the theoretical insights and exhaustive research of Mike Oliver and Colin Barnes will be obvious.

The first disability meeting I ever attended was a showing by Sisters against Disablement of a video on the Rehabilitation Act in 1984. It lit a slow-burning fuse within me, which has resulted in this book, and was part of the groundswell of disability activism which has now placed equal rights for disabled people firmly on the political agenda. It has been a long campaign but we are nearly there.

Table of Statutes

Table of Cases

UK

xiii

USA

Others

Table of Regulations and Statutory Instruments

Abbreviations

ACCD	American Coalition of Citizens with Disabilities
ADA	Americans with Disabilities Act
ADL	anti-discrimination legislation
BCODP	British Council of Organisations of Disabled People
BFOQ	bona fide occupational qualification
CORAD	Committee on the Restrictions against Disabled People
CPAG	Child Poverty Action Group
CRE	Commission for Racial Equality
CSDPA	Chronically Sick and Disabled Persons Act
DPTAC	Disabled People's Transport Advisory Committee
DPW	Department of Public Works (US)
DREDEF	Disability Rights and Education Fund (US)
DWA	Disability Working Allowance
EAT	Employment Appeal Tribunal
ECJ	European Court of Justice
EEOC	Equal Employment Opportunities Commission (US)
EOC	Equal Opportunities Commission
ERA	Equal Rights Amendment (US)
FEFC	Further Education Funding Council
HEW	Department of Health Education and Welfare (US)
ILM	Independent Living Movement (US)
IVB	Invalidity Benefit
NAACP	National Association for the Advancement of Colored People (US)
OCR	Office of Civil Rights (US)
OFCCP	Office of Federal Contract Compliance Programs (US)
OPCS	Office of Population Censuses and Surveys
PVA	Paralyzed Veterans of America
RAD	Royal Association in Aid of Deaf People
RADAR	Royal Association for Disability and Rehabilitation
RRA	Race Relations Act
SCPR	Social and Community Planning Research
SDA	Sex Discrimination Act
SEN	special educational needs
SPS	sheltered placement scheme
UPIAS	Union of the Physically Impaired against Segregation
VOADL	Voluntary Organisations for Anti-Discrimination Legislation
WARPATH	World Association to Remove Prejudice against the Handicapped

Introduction

This book looks back at how the law and discrimination have combined to produce disability; it also looks forward, raising the possibility that the law might 'change sides' and be used to counter discrimination and thereby deconstruct disability.

The idea that the law is not an impartial arbiter, but colludes with, and indeed itself perpetrates, discrimination may well seem less startling to the prospective readership of this book than the suggestion that discrimination 'causes' disability. To understand what is being suggested requires a re-examination of the accepted notions of both 'disability' and 'discrimination'.

The word discrimination is not one which has traditionally been associated with disabled people. The pervasive equation of disability with incapacity has meant that the inferior economic and social conditions of disabled people were seen as the natural consequences of their physical and mental 'impairments'. In this view treating disabled people differently is not the result of discrimination but the result of their 'special' needs because of their differences from the 'normal', able-bodied population. This treatment is seen as charitable, 'for their own good'.

Disabled people are challenging this interpretation: 'In our view it is society which disables ... impaired people. Disability is something which is imposed on top of our impairments by the way in which we are unnecessarily isolated and excluded from full participation in society.'[1]

This book argues that people possess physical and mental abilities in a broad spectrum from super-fit athlete, through someone with the aches and energy levels considered normal for their age group, to those people who are labelled as 'disabled'. Society has been constructed so as to meet the needs of only people within a narrow part of that spectrum. A dichotomy is thus set up between 'the able-bodied' who fit in, and 'the disabled', who don't.

Rather than seeing this exclusion as a consequence of the intrinsic characteristics of disabled people, in this volume it is viewed as the consequence of concrete social and historical processes. Chapter 1 briefly examines these processes, and the structural discrimination which they have created. In particular, the role of the modern welfare state in constructing a disabled identity is emphasised. This is then contrasted with the recent legislative initiatives in America, which have addressed the issue of disability from a rights based perspective.

The problematising of the existence and meaning of the differences ascribed to disabled people is at the heart of the disability movement and the theoretical analyses which it has developed. This issue is inevitably also at the heart of the debate as to whether anti-discrimination legislation, modelled on the laws banning sex and race discrimination, is appropriate to disabled people. Many theorists, whilst acknowledging the role that discrimination plays in disadvantaging disabled people, stress the dissimilarities with other forms of discrimination. In the words of one influential commentator: 'The most significant difference between the handicapped and other protected classes is that the condition which initially gives rise to the protected status may also affect their performance.'[2]

Not only does such a view continue to individualise the problems created for disabled people by a society structured so as to exclude them, it also embodies a very restricted view of the meaning of equality for other disadvantaged groups. Chapter 2 examines the feminist and anti-racist critiques of the dominant anti-discrimination paradigm (the 'formal equality' model) and argues that for other marginalised groups, as well as disabled people, 'the relevant differences have been, and always will be, those which keep [them] in their place.'[3]

A key goal of this book is to place disability within the broader spectrum of equal opportunities issues, and to stress the continuities between the experiences of disabled people and those of other so-called minority groups.

As well as problematising disability and discrimination, this book raises the question: 'What is the law?' The standard legal textbook treats the law in an abstract fashion, as a collection of statutes and legal decisions. Here, in contrast, the law is viewed as a social process, placing statutes and decisions within the context of the social forces which brought them into being and determining the impact which they will have.

This book is itself part of a social process, a product of the disability movement and a contribution to the campaign for a law to counter disability discrimination. Although such a law does not yet exist in Britain, it does exist in the United States, and a key goal of this book is to examine the lessons which can be drawn from the American experience. Chapters 3 and 4 examine the record of American disability legislation, on which a proposed British disability rights law has been modelled. In addition to looking at the practical potential of the law for removing barriers to disabled people's participation in society, I also consider its ideological impact in terms of its capacity for positively shaping public discourse, as well as for the empowerment of disabled people individually and collectively. It is argued that the American rights legislation's capacity for empowerment is particularly significant because of the dynamic inter-relationship of its rights discourse and the political process. The Rehabilitation Act, and still more the Americans with Disabilities Act, contain a powerful ideological message: that the chief problem con-fronting disabled people is social prejudice. As disabled people's self-image has been altered by this legislation, and by the process of fighting for its implementation, they have been empowered to become an effective political constituency, which is then able to press for stronger provisions and the effective mechanisms for enforcement which are so crucial to the success of anti-discrimination laws.

Thus an analysis of the different socio-political forces behind the legislation, which operate to improve and implement it, as well as those forces which seek to neutralise it, adds a crucial dimension to consid-erations of the likely effectiveness of the American legislation. The book's analysis therefore moves from a legal critique of the laws, via an overview of enforcement efforts, to a more historical and political analysis of the factors producing these laws. It assesses the potential of the legislation for overcoming any deficiencies in its drafting (whether the product of inadequate jurisprudential models or of com-promises in the legislative process) and achieving strong implementation.

As well as looking at the American experience with disability rights law, the experience of British sex and race discrimination laws are also reviewed. The object is to present a realistic picture of the obstacles which anti-discrimination legislation faces in the concrete legal and political conditions of Britain. Chapter 5 contrasts these conditions with those in America, whilst Chapter 6 looks at the consequences of these differences with regard to the impact of anti-discrimination laws in the areas of sex and race. The reasons why such laws have been less effective in Britain are summarised here, together with proposals for reform.

The final section of the book attempts to draw together these lessons from other experiences. Chapter 7 examines how a British Civil Rights Act for disabled people might be structured, taking into account the strengths and deficiencies of existing legislation. Chapter 8 details the campaign for such a law in Britain, and looks at the prospects for its success. It is suggested that just as the historical key to the current meaning of disability lies in the welfare state, so the current crisis and restructuring of it may present the key opportunity for a law which redefines the meaning of disability from a rights perspective.

1
Disability and Discrimination

The meaning of disability

To understand the meaning of 'disability' it is necessary to distinguish between an impairment and the disability which stems from it. An impairment is the functional limitation within the individual caused by physical, mental or sensory factors; a disability is the loss or limitation of opportunities to take part in the normal life of the community on an equal basis with others imposed on people with impairments by physical and social barriers.[1]

The vital feature of this definition of disability is that it distinguishes between the functional restrictions which are inherently associated with certain impairments (difficulty in walking, seeing, hearing, etc.) and those which stem from avoidable social restrictions. These restrictions may be social – refusal of entry to cinemas, clubs or employment – or environmental – stairs, poor lighting or lack of audio aids.

This book attempts to address the situations of all disabled people, whether they have physical impairments, learning difficulties, mental health problems, sensory impairments or long-term health problems such as cancer. It seeks to achieve this by focusing on the one experience which they all have in common – discrimination. Women, lesbians, gay men and black people with disabilities experience discrimination in differing ways, as indeed do people from differing social classes. This book does not attempt to capture this diversity of experience,[2] although a consideration of the lessons which disabled people can draw from the experiences of other 'marginalised' groups forms an integral part of the text.

The meaning of discrimination

Some instances of discrimination are blatant, for example where disabled people are refused admission to places purely because they are considered to be upsetting to other customers (still a very common occurrence). Other examples require us to expand our understanding of discrimination to include instances where it operates unintention-

1

ally and indirectly. This process has even more devastating effects than direct discrimination:

> [It] is built into the environment and into the very structure of our lives ... It is accepted that there should be flights of stairs that disabled people cannot manage, that many disabled children cannot go to ordinary schools or choose between the normal range of universities, that many disabled people cannot travel by public transport, ... [or] freely attend theatres or cinemas ... If for 'disabled' in that list one were to insert 'black' or 'female' one would immediately see the list as representing cases of discrimination ... if the only reason that a disabled person cannot get into a building is because it is part of a world that is constructed for non-disabled then it is just as much discrimination as if there was a notice on the door saying 'No disabled'.[3]

Discrimination is commonly understood as the prejudiced attitudes of individuals. Numerous studies show a combination of patronisation, pity and discomfort to be the dominant response of able-bodied people towards people with disabilities in Western societies, although fear, hatred and hostility are also prevalent.[4] It is difficult for able-bodied people to appreciate the full impact of such attitudes upon the lives of disabled people. Jenny Morris, in her book *Pride against Prejudice*, provides perhaps the most vivid account of the power of prejudice, both from her own experiences and through her interviews with other disabled women.[5] One woman lists the assumptions which underlie the actions of able-bodied people. Amongst these are:

> That we feel ugly, inadequate and ashamed of our disability.
> That our lives are a burden to us, barely worth living.
> That we crave to be 'normal' and 'whole'.
> That nothing can be gained from the experience.
> That we suffer and that any suffering is nasty, unjust and to be feared and retreated from.
> That we live naive and sheltered lives.
> That we 'never give up hope' of a cure.
> That those of us who ... require a carer to attend to our physical needs are helpless cabbages who don't do anything either and have nothing to give and who lead meaningless, empty lives.
> That we should put up with any inconvenience, discomfort or indignity in order to participate in 'normal' activities and events. And that this will somehow 'do us good'.[6]

It does not take any expertise in psychology to recognise the strength of these assumptions in our society, or just how undermining they are. Molly McIntosh's personal account of the impact of her facial scars on her life vividly illustrates this impact.

When I left school I did a typing course but found it difficult to get work. Typists were supposed to be attractive and cheerful and I was ugly and miserable. Even when I could get work, I just hated the way people reacted towards me when they first met me. In the end, my mother said I may as well stay at home and help her with the housework because she had got herself a part-time job. I started to enjoy my life more then.[7]

This is a woman whose 'disability' consists entirely of other people's attitudes, trapped in her own home as she limits her excursions into the outside world to the maximum possible extent.

Clare Robson's disability caused her to experience shaking in one side of her body, and she used a cane to walk. She relates how strangers frequently came up to her in the street to ask what was wrong. 'If I told them, they would say "Oh how awful, there's no cure for that, is there?"' She comments: 'It's pity that motivates that kind of reaction, not empathy. And also it's voyeurism.'[8]

These experiences are all too 'normal' for disabled people. Jenny Morris comments: 'It is not only physical limitations that restrict us to our homes and those whom we know. It is the knowledge that each entry into the public world will be dominated by stares, condescension, by pity and by hostility.'[9]

The stigmatising effects of disability are compounded by the barriers presented by a world designed for the able-bodied. Hahn, commenting on American social policy, poses the issue in this manner:

The existence of an environment which is inaccessible to large numbers of people raises some troubling but unavoidable questions about the normative assumptions which a nation might impose upon the physical capacities of its citizens. In order to pursue what most people would consider an acceptable or tolerable life, for example, should individuals be expected to walk? To run? To see and hear clearly? To speak articulately?[10]

I would argue that these questions represent political choices. Having created an exclusionary and segregated society, how far is the able-bodied majority prepared to go to reshape that society so that it includes the whole spectrum of abilities? A brief consideration of the position of disabled people with regard to transport, housing and employment will illustrate the extent of the problem.

Transport
'Public' transport provides a classic illustration of the devastating effect of designing facilities for a narrow range of physical abilities. The official British advisory committee on disability and public transport,

the Disabled People's Transport Advisory Committee (DPTAC), estimated in its 1989 report that between 10 and 12 per cent of the population were unable to access the public transport system adequately.[11] Buses are inaccessible to many people with mobility restrictions, most obviously to wheelchair users, and fail to incorporate into their design those features which would improve their use by people with sensory impairments. Similarly, few long-distance coaches can be used by wheelchair occupants. Indeed the steep stairs on most coaches make them inaccessible to many people with mobility impairments. In 1990 only nine out of 800 National Express coaches had kneeling mechanisms to make them accessible to people in wheelchairs.[12]

DPTAC has produced a list of specifications required to improve the use of buses.[13] It is important to note that these design features would substantially improve the design of buses for able-bodied people as well – particularly for children and people with heavy shopping. In London only 500 out of 5,000 buses have such modifications.[14]

In the railway service, travelling in the guard's van is still a common experience for wheelchair users, and few trains have accessible toilets. The vast majority of stations are inaccessible to the disabled, and British Rail itself warns disabled travellers against using the hundreds of unstaffed stations.[15]

The effects of designing public transport facilities in such a way as to make them unusable by many disabled people is to imprison many in their homes, and to increase the expense, discomfort and difficulties of journeys for many others. This in turn restricts their ability to participate in community life, and in particular to work.

The remedies put forward, once the consequences of exclusion from 'public' transport began to be appreciated, have served only to avoid the issue, leaving public transport's inaccessibility unchallenged. Various state benefits seek to compensate for the extra costs incurred by those with restricted mobility, caused in part by the inaccessibility of public transport. The principal state benefit is the mobility component of the Disability Living Allowance, and in addition specific schemes exist to compensate for the extra costs of travelling to work, education and/or training. These benefits are invariably inadequate for meeting the additional costs, and have complicated eligibility requirements which make them difficult to claim. Moreover, receiving state benefits attracts stigma in this society. For this reason, and because of inadequate information, many eligible disabled people fail to claim.

The second approach is the provision of segregated transport services. Many local authorities provide Dial-A-Ride services. However, these are universally inferior to mainstream services, being under-funded and grossly limited in scope. Users have to book rides well in advance, services operate at limited times and restrictions are often made on the frequency of rides.

These illustrate the two classic state responses to disability – welfare provision and segregation. Neither of these approaches is an adequate substitute for a public transport system designed to be used by all members of the public.

Housing

The situation with regard to housing for disabled people is equally desperate. Despite the fact that there are 4.25 million people with mobility impairments in Britain, there are only 80,000 accessible homes.[16]

Once again this is the result of services being designed and provided in such a way as to meet the needs of only a narrow spectrum of their potential users. Historically, disabled people have been forced to live in segregated institutions, and to this day the construction of separate housing schemes designed for those with 'special' needs perpetuates this approach. Once again, this policy means that the mainstream of provision continues to exclude disabled people.

The concept of adaptable housing has been articulated as a more progressive response to the needs of disabled people. Its principles are succinctly stated by Rachel Hurst, a leading disability activist:

I believe that the most effective way in which we are going to achieve our goal of removing the discrimination we face will be through the inclusion of disabled people's needs in general housing and building legislation and regulations ... Why do we have to move if we're disabled? ... And why can't we visit our friends and neighbours? I am not suggesting that all housing should be built to what are known as 'wheelchair standards', but that homes have level thresholds, wide doorways, plugs at reasonable height, and a loo at the entrance level. This ... is what most people want ... Particularly those with young children and prams, or elderly people. That is most of the population.[17]

Such mobility or adaptable housing, whilst not itself immediately suitable for occupation (as opposed to visiting) by wheelchair users is easily adaptable for such use – merely by adding a stair lift. The extra cost of such new buildings is negligible compared to the price of adapting buildings later on.

Houses are used by a succession of occupants, over different stretches of their life cycles, and should be suited to this purpose.[18] Adaptable housing is important, not only because it is a practical way to increase the usable proportion of housing stock, but also because it breaks away from the notions of ghettoised 'special needs' housing for the minority, and recognises that a wide variety of people benefit from a friendlier environment.

Employment

The devastating effects of social attitudes and environmental barriers are testified to by the figures for the unemployment and under employment of disabled people. In Britain the official unemployment rate for disabled people is 20 per cent, compared to 9 per cent for able-bodied people.[19] In fact the actual unemployment rate is much higher. Two-thirds of disabled people do not work, and a survey by the Office of Population Censuses and Surveys found that half of these wanted to work, given the right circumstances.[20]

As for under employment, disabled people in full-time occupations earn on average two-thirds the wages of able-bodied workers.[21] Government research into problems encountered in employment showed that they are also more likely to be employed in manual or unskilled occupations than able-bodied workers: 12 per cent of disabled workers are in professional or managerial positions compared to 21 per cent of non-disabled workers; 31 per cent of disabled workers are in low skilled manual occupations compared to 21 per cent of non-disabled workers.[22]

To an extent this reflects the poorer education which children with disabilities tend to receive. However, the majority of people with impairments become disabled during the course of their lives. For these people, disability frequently leads to the loss of a job. Only one-third of people who were in employment at the time they became disabled retained their jobs.[23] A survey carried out by the Association of Disabled Professionals found that a third of respondents felt that their intellectual abilities and professional training had been under-utilised since they became disabled.[24]

The 'common sense' explanation for these statistics is that they reflect restrictions on work capacity caused by the physical or mental impairments of disabled people. However, this is contradicted by the evidence. There are numerous studies which ask employers to evaluate the work performance of disabled employees.[25] All of these reveal a high level of satisfaction. Perhaps the most extensive survey was carried out by the US Department of Labor in 1948.[26] This study examined the records of 48,000 disabled and able-bodied workers, and concluded that in terms of productivity, safety and absenteeism disabled workers ranked equally with able-bodied ones. The only difference was that a greater number of disabled workers lost their jobs, the result of able-bodied workers moving back into the jobs which they had held before the Second World War (a process very similar to that involving female war workers who also lost their jobs in 'male' industries once the war ended).

Amongst employers with no experience of employing disabled workers the myths of poor work-capacity and sickness problems remain strong. A 1993 survey of employers' attitudes and actions with regard

to disabled workers found that 42 per cent of the companies interv
employed no disabled people.[27] One of the most frequently
reasons for this was that there were no suitable jobs for disabled
workers within the organisation. Since the survey had deliberately
included a spread of sizes of firms, from under ten employees to over
5,000, it is highly unlikely that the respondents truly had no posts which
could be filled by anyone with any degree of disability. The researcher
comments: 'Many of the perceived difficulties are associated with
somewhat stereotypical views of the range of disabilities likely to be
encountered.'[28] Thus, one of the commonest explanations for the
unsuitability of the work was its 'physical nature'. And yet, as we have
seen, a higher proportion of disabled people work in manual jobs
than do able-bodied people. A government commissioned survey
found that another common reason given by employers for not
employing disabled people was the lack of accessible premises.[29] These
employers equate disability with wheelchairs, and yet only 5 per cent
of disabled people use wheelchairs.

To an extent some of these 'reasons' are simply an excuse for discrimination. Some employers are blatant in their attitudes: 6 per cent
of employers in the same survey said that they would not employ
disabled people under any circumstances.[30] A survey of disabled
solicitors found that 21 per cent thought that their careers would be
affected by prejudice. A further 8 per cent said that they experienced
'appearance problems'. 'What clients would think' was the commonest
reason for rejection given by potential employers.[31]

Physiotherapists were interviewed about the suitability of disabled
people for their profession.[32] Twenty per cent thought that people with
controlled epilepsy should not be allowed to work as physiotherapists;
22 per cent thought that people with histories of depression should
not be physiotherapists; and a further 17 per cent thought that people
with severe facial deformities were unsuitable.

If the stereotyping and underestimation of disabled people's abilities
is one-half of the equation, the other half is a distorted sense of what
abilities are required to carry out a job. A previous survey of employers'
attitudes[33] found that 65 per cent thought that being able to climb
stairs was 'vital for work in management'; a further 75 per cent thought
that good eyesight was 'vital' for managerial work. Thirty-one per cent
stated that the ability to walk fairly long distances was vital for a
career as a business professional.

Many disabled people do not require any 'special' provisions, but
the working environment does create real problems for some people
with disabilities. For example, in the same survey of disabled solicitors,
21 per cent thought that their careers would be adversely affected by
access problems.[34]

It is not only the physical working environment which creates problems for disabled people. People whose disabilities entail fatigue and or pain may require flexible working hours or part-time employment.[35] Able-bodied women, seeking to combine their role in the home with paid work, often require the same sort of flexibility in working arrangements. As we will see, the failure of the 'standard' working environment to meet these needs creates structural disadvantages for women which the anti-discrimination laws have found hard to counter. Disabled women are not surprisingly far more likely to require flexible working arrangements, and are thus at a double disadvantage.

Just as buildings, machinery and working hours have been designed to suit able-bodied men, so the division of tasks within a team of workers also tends to be premised on all the workers being able-bodied. Where an individual's disability makes it difficult for them to carry out a particular task, it is often possible to reorganise the tasks within a team, without undue disruption. For example, a deaf person in an office may not be able to use the telephone, and this role could be exchanged for other administrative roles within the team. In the Social and Community Planning Research survey 28 per cent of disabled people reported that they would require some flexibility with work tasks.[36] (In addition, 9 per cent required rest periods during the day; and 6 per cent needed assistance all or most of the time. This survey is likely to exaggerate the extent of requirements amongst disabled people, as the researchers restricted their enquiries from the beginning to those who are 'occupationally handicapped', the 3 per cent of the population whose disability has most impact on their work performance. In particular, the survey underrepresents people with mental health problems or learning disabilities.)

It is important to recognise that such reorganisations of tasks to suit the capabilities of workers takes place amongst able-bodied people all the time. Rearranging roles to take into account a person's disability should be seen as an extension of this process rather than as an exceptional requirement. Indeed, all the structural barriers discussed above are the consequences of designing environments to exclude disabled people.

Finally, discriminatory provision in other areas affects disabled people's chances in employment. Thirty-nine per cent of disabled people in the above survey reported that their journey was more tiring, and 9 per cent said it cost more. A further 5 per cent worked from home, in part due to transport difficulties.[37]

The construction of disability

The policy question of how broad a spectrum of abilities structures should be designed to cater for becomes all the more pertinent when we recognise that the sharp dichotomy between able-bodied and disabled, present in popular opinion and theoretical texts alike, is a social myth. To understand the full operation of discrimination on disabled people's lives we need to extend our understanding of that process to include the socio-economic and political forces which shape not only our attitudes towards disability, but also the very meaning of that term. In a very real sense our society disables individuals by constructing a disabled identity into which individuals are fitted.

Functional abilities are in fact possessed by people in a broad range, from super-fit athletes, through people with aches and pains that we associate as 'normal' for their age group, to those with limitations that we have traditionally labelled as 'disabled'. A study of functional impairments reported that 14 per cent of all adults in Britain living in private households (6.2 million persons) have difficulty in performing one or more basic physical activities such as seeing, hearing, speaking, walking, using stairs, lifting or carrying.[38] This survey found that 1.7 million had trouble seeing words in newspapers, even with glasses; 2.5 million had trouble hearing a normal conversation; and 1.2 million had trouble making their speech understood.

These figures graphically illustrate the falsity of our conception of 'the disabled' as a separate category (the 'Other'). In fact, definitions of disability are socially based, depending on our expectations of the abilities which an average member of society will possess, and varying with age and sex. Intelligence Quotient (IQ) and the labelling of 'mental handicapped' (in place of this stigmatising term I will refer in this book to people with learning difficulties), for example, are based on the statistical concept of the 'standard deviation from the norm', which means that they are defined in reference to the scores achieved in tests by the majority of the population. 'Mental handicap' is thus not an absolute term, but a socially relative one, reflecting as it does an expectation of those mental capacities which are required for 'normal' functioning in society:

> Thus labelling people as mentally ill or handicapped is an indicator of what can be tolerated within mainstream settings. The limbo in which people so labelled exist effectively insulates the male world of work from failure, distress, illness and vulnerability just as the marginalisation of women and children within the shrinking nuclear family have protected it from the demands of personal relationships and dependence.[39]

Similarly the labels 'blind' or 'deaf' are relative ones, based on the percentage of 'full' vision or hearing which a person possesses. To be 'legally' blind or deaf does not necessarily mean that an individual lacks all visual or aural capacity.

Labels such as 'blind' or 'deaf' or 'mentally handicapped' also simplify, in order to measure, a very complex mixture of abilities which we then term 'sight' or 'hearing' or 'intelligence'. Thus, for example, vision consists of a collection of different functions – seeing at a distance and close up, seeing in bright light or dark, peripheral vision, ability to distinguish colours.

The above comments relate to the classic stereotypes of disability – deafness, blindness, permanent physical impairments, learning difficulties – but they also apply to the much broader definition used in this book. Many disabilities are the result of long-term illnesses, often of a fluctuating nature. Here again the question can be posed, at what point does 'ill-health' become 'disability'? A spectrum of health is clearly present within our society. Respiratory difficulties and 'bad backs' can both be immensely disabling, but are also impairments which are present in many members of the population in a mild form. Doyal's comments on the social construction of definitions of health and illness are pertinent: 'Health is usually defined as "fitness" to undertake whatever would be expected of someone in a particular social position.'[40]

Similar considerations apply to mental illness. (Although mental illness is not included in the everyday understanding of disability, people with mental health problems are very significantly represented within state disability programmes, and very much a part of the disability movement.) There is a substantial literature questioning the normative nature of good mental health[41] and MIND, the national mental health charity, has calculated that one in ten people have a diagnosis of mental illness at any one time.[42]

The shifting meaning of disability

Precisely because of their normative nature, classifications of disability have varied historically. In part these historical variations result from shifts in technology and the social conditions in which that technology is disseminated. An illustration of how technological and social conditions underlie, and are obscured by, our definitions of disability is provided by the example of visually impaired people who by wearing glasses can possess a 'normal' range of vision. Often these people would be unable to read or distinguish objects without their visual aids. Yet they will not be considered 'disabled', both because this impairment is sufficiently widespread not to be stigmatised and because in our society such corrective aids are readily available.

The technological level of society can reduce disabilities by 'curing' physical impairments or by reducing their impact on the individual's ability to function – as spectacles have done. However it can also, paradoxically, increase them. Medical advances can increase the numbers of disabled people, prolonging the lives of people who would previously have died. Less positively, society can disable more individuals by increasing the level at which individuals are expected to function in society, and hence magnifying the disabling effects of impairments. One example of this process is the invention of the telephone, which has had a detrimental impact on the ability of deaf people to function socially. On a broader level, disabled theorists such as Victor Finklestein[43] and Mike Oliver[44] argue that the industrial revolution and the introduction of mass production operated to exclude disabled people, and that, more recently, technological developments, particularly computerisation, have created the potential for the integration of disabled people into mainstream economic activity.

Disability as a political category

So far we have assumed that 'disability' is a social category imposed on individuals who have 'impairments'. Gillian Fulcher problematises the concept of 'disability' a stage further, by questioning the causal equation 'impairment therefore disability'. She defines disability as a 'political and procedural category' and stresses that the existence of an impairment is not necessarily the determining cause of an individual being labelled as 'disabled'.[45] This is clearly illustrated in the subject area of her analysis, 'special needs education'. Her approach does not assume the presence of a pre-existing category of children with impairments, as do many writers on the subject, who then confine their analyses to how this group of children is treated in policy terms. Instead, she examines how the creation of such a category then produces processes by which children are recruited to fill it. Squibb argues similarly: 'It is this process [of definition] which produces the special child rather than anything which the child may or may not have within him or her.'[46]

It is relatively easy to recognise the truth of this with regard to 'behavioural problems', which are more obviously the product of social labelling. But with physical impairments too there can be strong disagreements about whether, for example, a partially sighted child, a deaf child or a child with cerebral palsy should attract these labels. Examining the official figures for 'handicapped' children from 1961 to 1976 Squibb notes a 195 per cent increase in those with partial hearing; children with epilepsy increased by 59 per cent, and those with 'speech defects' by a staggering 1,332 per cent. Squibb suggests that this may in part reflect increasingly sensitive diagnostic techniques, but also recognises the importance of understanding the structural forces which propelled the development of techniques and applied them to schoolchildren. Why was it important to schools to label more children?

The reason generally put forward for identifying more precisely the physical, mental and emotional conditions of pupils is to enable their needs to be more adequately catered for. Critical theorists, particularly disabled ones, question this justification, suggesting that the labelling of pupils has much more to do with the needs of the system than with those of individual pupils:

> The initial development of segregated special education was a consequence of the vested interest of the ordinary school sector who were concerned that their payment-by-results benefits would be adversely affected by the presence of a variety of demanding and disruptive pupils. Subsequent trends were shaped by the growing power of newly developing professions, notably school doctors, teachers, educational administrators and psychologists.[47]

In consequence a number of new categories for disabled children grew in the 1960s: 'aphasic', 'dyslexic', 'autistic', 'psychologically crippled' and 'socially handicapped', all of which children were recommended for 'special' education.

Another strand of explanation points to the functioning of such labels as a form of social control. This is again most evident in relation to those labelled as having 'behavioural problems', but also applies to children with learning difficulties. Thus, black children and boys generally are more likely to be labelled as 'educationally sub-normal'. Barton and Tomlinson suggest that the labelling of children with disabilities is part of a broader process of controlling deviant sectors of the school population. They argue that disabled children are controlled 'as just another problem group in society, making them productive if possible, dealing with them as cheaply as possible if not, and legitimating them as unemployable in a time of high unemployment.'[48]

If education can be a crucial process in constructing an individual's identity as disabled, the procedures and institutions of the welfare state are even more central to producing the category 'disabled'. The capacity which the state benefit system has to construct the meaning of a disabled identity is clearly illustrated by a recent House of Lords decision. The case involved a severely disabled woman who lived at home with her parents and sought to claim severe disability premium under the Social Security Act 1986. However, the regulations[49] provided that claimants were not entitled to the premium where they lived with 'non-dependants'. These regulations had been made under the Secretary of State's power to specify 'the circumstances in which persons are to be treated as being or as not being severely disabled'. Ms Foster appealed on the grounds that the Secretary of State had exceeded his powers of regulation, since the 1987 regulations did not relate to the degree of disability, but to the social circumstances of an individual. The House of Lords dismissed her appeal, on the basis that when defining the category of persons who would be regarded as severely disabled the

Secretary of State was entitled to take into account 'circumstances relevant to the disabled person's needs'.[50] This is confirmation from an unlikely quarter that disability is in essence a social rather than a medical concept.

A number of writers have described the process by which the institutions of the welfare state induce disabled people to assume the roles which are considered appropriate for their status. Scott, for example, vividly describes the process by which blind men have their identities formed through their interaction with welfare agencies.[51] Liggett notes how even the conservative defenders of current disability programmes inadvertently acknowledge the power of this process:

> Even Howards et al. show how disability programmes are active producers of disability. Widows who do not meet the specified criteria of the Social Security Administration are 'for practical purposes "non-widows"'. What they don't say and what symbolic interactionist studies record is that women who do meet the qualifications are encouraged by their engagement with the system to constitute themselves as widows in its terms.[52]

Historical production of disability

As well as powerfully influencing the construction of individual disabled identities, the welfare state is also central to the historical development of the disabled category. Thus Deborah Stone argues persuasively that 'what seems to us so obvious now – that there is a state of being called "disabled" which is clearly different from the normal state of being and which requires special treatment – is a fairly modern perception.'[53]

Whilst the stigmatisation of impairments is a cross-cultural and trans-historical phenomenon,[54] the distinctive category 'the disabled' is the product of recent (nineteenth- and twentieth-century) development both in the forms of economic production (industrial capitalism) and of the social relations of production and reproduction.

There have been no detailed historical studies of the effects of changes in the modes and relations of economic production upon the integration of disabled people into the labour market. Finklestein theorises that in pre-industrial society the economy was based in agriculture and small-scale crafts, organised around the family as a unit of production. The great majority of disabled people were able to contribute to the production process in this phase.[55] However, the rise of capitalist industrialisation together with large-scale production processes excluded many from the production process:

> The speed of factory work, the enforced discipline, the time keeping and production norms – all these were a highly unfavourable change

from the slower, more self-determined and flexible methods of work into which many handicapped people had been integrated.[56]

With the rise of capitalism, alongside the changes in the productive process which excluded many disabled people from the workforce, went changes in social relations that were at least as important. In pre-capitalist society individuals depended on the family unit for their needs, and in return contributed what they could to the production process (or perhaps supplemented the family income by begging). Under the capitalist waged economy, individuals would only be allowed access to the means of production if, in exchange for wages, they produced the maximum amount of profit for the owner of the means of production:

> The 'body' – the body of individuals and the body of populations – appears as the bearer of new variables, not merely between the scarce and the numerous, the submissive and the restive, rich and poor, healthy and sick, strong and weak, but also between the more or less utilizable, more or less amenable to profitable investment, those with greater or lesser prospects of survival, death and illness, and with more or less capacity to be usefully trained.[57]

Michael Oliver quotes this passage by Foucault to point out the significance of the ideological shifts produced by capitalism, and in particular the importance to the new order of 'able-bodied' workers with the ability to operate the new machines and a willingness to submit to the new factory disciplines.[58]

Doyal also emphasises the role which the emergence of capitalist industry played in shaping people's understanding of the nature of health.

> The defining of health and illness in a functional way is an important example of how a capitalist system defines people primarily as producers – as forces of production. It is concerned with their 'fitness' in an instrumental sense ... In defining health and illness in this way, the medical model limits people's own expectations of what it is to be healthy ... But under capitalism, health is also defined in an individualistic way. It is always individuals who become sick, rather than social, economic or environmental factors which cause them to become so.[59]

The welfare state and disabled identity

These changes in the productivity of disabled people put a strain on the ability of families to provide for disabled members. Increasingly the resolution of this problem was state provision. Deborah Stone argues:

> The very notion of disability is fundamental to the architecture of the welfare state; it is something like a keystone that allows the other supporting structures of the welfare state, and, in some senses the economy at large, to stay in place.[60]

Stone suggests that the concept of disability has been used to resolve the issue of distributive justice. This issue is created by the presence within the modern world of two distributive systems – one of which distributes on the basis of waged labour and the other on the basis of need. There is a potential conflict between these two systems since if people can acquire goods through the need system they will not need to engage in waged work; this has been termed the 'disincentive' problem of welfare benefits. (It has been noted in this context that: 'Women often share this ambiguous economic status since they are rarely able to support themselves and their dependants; the more needs they are responsible for meeting the less likely they are to be in the market place at all.')[61]

This conflict has historically been resolved by the creation of rigid categories of need – the elderly, children, the disabled – to determine who will be allowed to claim public assistance. These categories are premised on exclusion from the labour market. Hence, disability becomes synonymous with dependence and inability to work. This is perhaps the most powerful impact of the welfare state on the meaning of disability, but it had a number of other powerful ideological consequences, whose impact is heightened by the 'discursive practices'[62] which accompany them.

Radical interpretations of the welfare state have seen it as both fulfilling the need of the ruling class for social control, and as the product of struggles between competing factions within the ruling class, and their discursive practices.[63] In the case of disabled people these forces have meant that institutionalisation, segregation, medicalisation and the production of dependency have been the dominant characteristics of their treatment by the welfare institutions.

Institutions

Historically 'welfare provision' for disabled people has taken the form of segregated institutions. Dehumanising per se, where abuses occur it can involve gross understaffing, physical abuse and neglect, medical experimentation, the use of solitary confinement and physical restraints.

Rothman argues that an important function of this progress of institutionalisation was as a form of social control.[64] Initially most disabled people who entered institutions were forced into workhouses. These served a policing role between the two distributive systems described by Stone, waged labour and need, part of a broader deterrent aimed at able-bodied malingerers. 'The workhouse was intended to be so unpleasant and unattractive that no one who could possibly work would choose to enter it instead.'[65]

From its initiation by the Poor Law Amendment Act 1834, the Poor Law Commission decreed that the 'aged and infirm' (the 'deserving poor') should be treated separately from the able-bodied poor. This category eventually became sub-divided into four specific categories – the 'sick', the 'insane', 'defectives' (such as people with sensory impairments, people with epilepsy and those defined as 'mentally sub-normal') and the 'aged and infirm'. Each was treated differently, and increasingly through specialised institutions.[66] For example, the Mental Deficiency Act 1913 established a network of institutions or 'colonies' for people with learning difficulties. The treatment of those labelled as mentally ill probably best exemplifies this process:

> Up to the second half of the eighteenth century, mentally disturbed people were not categorised separately from other indigent people, and were very seldom cared for in segregated institutions. By the mid-nineteenth century, however, the insane found themselves incarcerated in a specialised, bureaucratically organised, state-supported asylum system which isolated them both physically and symbolically from the larger society.[67]

At the end of the nineteenth century the rationale for these institutions was that they protected the disabled from society. In the early twentieth century, with the rise of the eugenicist movement, people with disabilities became seen as the source of a wide variety of social ills, so that the new rationale for exclusion was to protect society from 'the disabled'. Thus, the trend towards segregation in specialised institutions gathered force throughout the twentieth century, so that by its peak in 1954 there were 148,000 patients in public asylums.

Throughout the 1960s and 1970s there was increasing recognition of the damage caused by institutionalisation. However, although the rhetoric changed the practice was slow to follow. Thus, whilst the idea that people with learning difficulties could live outside large hospitals was central to the Mental Health Act 1959, this legislative change brought little practical change. 'In practice, the large hospitals continued to be the main providers of accommodation outside the family home.'[68] Harrison discerns a similiar contradiction between theory and practice for young physically disabled adults since 1970: 'Despite the greater emphasis on community care during that time, the total number of occupied places has significantly increased'.[69]

The impact of institutionalisation extends beyond the large numbers of disabled people who have had first-hand experience of it. It has also had a powerful impact on how disabled people are seen by society, intensifying the stigma associated with impairments, and contributing to the broader social processes of segregation and medicalisation.

Segregation

Segregation persists as one of the fundamental modes of control utilised by the state with regard to disabled people. The impact of segregation upon the lives of disabled people cannot be overestimated. The lack of contact with non-disabled people undoubtedly contributes to the fear, embarrassment and powerful stereotypes which we have seen characterise able-bodied people's reactions to disabled people. It has also intensified the tendency to construct the environment exclusively for the use of non-disabled people, thus in turn accentuating the forces of segregation. The end result is that modern society has been built upon the basis of excluding disabled people and the range of human needs they represent. Frank Bowe describes the situation most eloquently:

> For 200 years we have designed a nation for the average, normal, able-bodied majority, little realizing that millions cannot enter many of our buildings, ride our subways and our buses, enjoy our educational and recreational programs and facilities and use our communication systems ... We have said for 200 years and say anew every day that we do not wish to see disabled people ... We do not wish to be reminded of their needs or their desires to live in the world. We prefer these people to be sequestered safely in secluded institutions – and they have been. We prefer them to remain second class citizens – and they are. Most of all we stubbornly refuse to recognize that the problems that disabled people face are not theirs alone ... Disabled people have been out of the mainstream of American life for 200 years and these years have seen the construction of modern American society. So that now when they are coming back into our society the barriers that they face are enormous.[70]

Medicalisation

A key set of discursive practices influencing the formation of the welfare state is those of the medical profession; indeed its rising power was closely associated with the growth of the welfare state:

> Throughout the nineteenth century, medicine developed rapidly as a new and powerful science ... Medical ideas, and the activities and pronouncements of doctors, were a very powerful social force ... This power arose from the ideological importance of medicine in defining

and justifying new modes of social and economic organisation as well as from the growing significance of medical practice itself as a mechanism of social control.[71]

The medicalisation of social 'problems' as a form of control has been powerfully analysed by writers such as Foucault and Illich.[72] By 'medicalisation' I mean the perception that disability is first and foremost a medical problem of individuals, with the corresponding power that this gives to the medical profession over disabled people's lives. Whilst medical intervention can be entirely appropriate, for example in the treatment of a medical condition or the diagnosis of an impairment, it undoubtedly extends to a ridiculous degree. Mike Oliver gives the following examples:

> Doctors are also involved in assessing driving ability, prescribing wheelchairs, determining the allocation of financial benefits, selecting educational provision and measuring work capacities and potential ... in none of these cases is it immediately obvious that medical training and qualifications make doctors the most appropriate persons to be involved.[73]

The medical profession came to hold great power over disabled people's lives, both within institutions and outside them, through their function as gate-keepers of the welfare state.

Dependency

The post-1945 welfare state became more paternalistic, losing some of its harshness. Undoubtedly, many of the reforms had a progressive impact. Thus, the Education Act 1944 stated that every child should receive suitable education (although those classified as 'severely subnormal' were not to receive education, but merely 'treatment'), and that special educational 'treatment' should be provided for those who needed it: The National Health Services Act 1948 gave local authority health departments the power to provide any medical aids needed to enable disabled people to live at home; and the National Assistance Act 1948 required local authorities to provide residential facilities for disabled people.

In the legislation establishing the new welfare system the key concept used when referring to disabled people was that of 'need'. However, control over defining the needs of disabled people, and stipulating how these needs would be met, was placed in the hands of professionals, often medical professionals. This system is based on the assumption that disabled people are incapable of running their own lives, and forces them to become passive recipients of those services which other people think they ought to have. 'Above all else, assessment of needs is an exercise in power ... And there have been numerous studies which show that clients are very unhappy about the way professional assessments of all kinds have distorted or denied their needs.'[74] The system is dominated by the interests of the professionals who run it, rather than catering for the needs of disabled people themselves, with the effect that needs remain unmet or inappropriately met. The net result of the welfare state is that disabled people are denied opportunities to live autonomously. To an extent this stems from the state agencies' desire to control the level of resources, but it is also the product of less rational impulses, and in particular of deep-rooted beliefs that disabled people are lesser humans.

A different approach: the US experience

Disabled people have, through their own, increasingly militant organisations, been formulating their own understanding of the 'problems' confronting them in society. These form a striking contrast with the pattern of provision, and underlying assumptions, of the British welfare state. In particular, the disability movement takes as the starting point for its analysis and demands the need for action to halt the disabling processes described above, rather than merely alleviating the effects. Such action fundamentally involves taking power from professionals and claiming it for disabled people themselves. Policies must be based on a non-medical understanding of the nature of disability and must attack both segregation and discrimination. In formulating its demands the British disability movement has been powerfully influenced and inspired by developments in the US.

The first American legislation to recognise the existence of discrimination against disabled people, and take steps to counter it, was the Rehabilitation Act 1973. Provisions in this Act banned discrimination against disabled people in federally funded programmes, including transport and higher education. It also banned employment discrimination by the federal government or by businesses contracting with the Federal government. The Americans with Disabilities Act 1990 substantially broadened the anti-discrimination mandate contained in the 1973 Act, to include private businesses as employers and providers of services to the public. These two laws will be considered in considerable detail in Chapters 3 and 4.

Two other pieces of legislation based on the right of disabled people to non-discriminatory and integrated services were passed in the intervening years. The Education of All Handicapped Children Act 1975 mandated free, appropriate public education for all children with disabilities. It requires them to be educated in the 'least restrictive environment', with their non-disabled peers to the maximum extent appropriate. The Federal Fair Housing Amendment of 1988 added disabled people as a group protected from discrimination in housing. This was the first time that the anti-discrimination principle regarding disabled people was extended to the private sector. The law mandates accessibility standards for all new housing construction for multi-family dwellings and ensures that disabled people are able to adapt their dwelling places to meet their needs.

It is useful to understand how the United States legislation came to be based on the concept of rights rather than the British emphasis on needs. Up to the Rehabilitation Act, the American legislative approach to disability had been broadly similar to the British one outlined above. It is no accident that the breakthrough legislation providing civil rights for disabled people was contained in the Rehabilitation Act 1973. This had been America's 'progressive response' to disability in the twentieth Century.

Richard Scotch's definitive history, *From Goodwill to Civil Rights* (on which much of the account below is based) argues:

> The concept of rehabilitation was at the core of the ideology of the emerging American welfare state ... However the idea of individual rehabilitation was to be seen in subsequent years as inadequate. Rehabilitation would enable an individual to participate in social institutions only to the extent that the individual's participation was welcome and not dependent on disruptive accommodation.[75]

(As in Britain, the other dominant strand in American legislative provision for disabled people was income support, first provided by the Social Security Act 1935, amended and extended in 1956 and again in 1972. I referred above to Deborah Stone's analysis which locates the development of the category 'disabled' in the need to resolve the conflict between a distribution system based on need, and one operating through waged labour, and I will return to this issue in considering the causal factors behind the Americans with Disabilities Act.)

Growth of the disability movement

A crucial factor behind the shift which occurred in legislative provisions from these welfarist models to ones which focused on rights against discrimination was the growth of a unified and increasingly militant disability movement. The two greatest barriers to the formation of such a movement were the diversity of disabled people and the historical tendency of organisations with a charitable emphasis to be formed by able-bodied people. Although organisations of (rather than 'for') disabled people have a long history, nevertheless the National Federation of the Blind (founded in 1940) was the exception rather than the rule with its strong civil rights emphasis. Disabled people historically have been divided by their diverse physical and mental conditions, as well as being distributed amongst different classes and cultural backgrounds. Although, as we have seen, they do share a common history of exclusion, until recently:

> this exclusion has impeded them from developing a common identity or literally meeting on common ground. Interaction amongst disabled people sometimes reflects the stigmatization of disability practiced by the rest of society. In such instances, disabled individuals deliberately distance themselves from each other or make invidious distinctions between good and bad handicaps, rather than seeking to develop social ties on the basis of common experience.[76]

This situation began to change in the 1960s and early 1970s:

> Following in the wake of the Black power, feminist and other social movements of the 1960s, which also stressed a positive self-image rooted in the collective identity of an excluded group demanding greater participation, increasing numbers of disabled people embraced activism and the creation of community.[77]

Besides the influence of other protest movements, Scotch also credits the developments of technologies which enabled disabled people to lead a more independent life, and the increasing number of elderly people in America, many of whom have disabilities, with contributing to this radicalisation process. Indeed, the Grey Panther movement of elderly Americans itself contributed to the lobbying process.

The birth of the modern disability movement is generally located in the emergence of the Independent Living Movement (ILM) in Berkeley in the early 1970s. This developed the concept of the social causes of disability, and attempted to change the situation by setting up alternative kinds of service provision controlled by disabled people themselves. This development coincided with the founding of activist groups around the country, such as Judy Heuman's Disabled in Action in New York. This militant, cross-disability group focused on countering the process by which society disables the individual, and soon spread to several other cities. In 1974 the American Coalition of Citizens with Disabilities (ACCD) was founded, a cross-disability coalition of groups which was to provide a powerful focus for political action.

The most powerful disability groups, such as the Paralyzed Veterans of America (PVA) and the ACCD, were very much influenced by the civil rights struggle. This provided both a model for understanding the position of disabled people (just as women's and gay liberation were influenced by this political understanding of their situation) and strategies of action, such as sit-ins and other symbolic actions, for mobilising latent support within a constituency as well as amongst the general public.

The impact of the Vietnam war was also crucial, both in the influence of the anti-war movement and because of the disabled veterans' contribution to the disability movement.

> Disabled Vietnam veterans who returned home from an unpopular war viewed themselves as suffering the same kind of discrimination and ostracism that minorities had endured and sought to overcome. Having responded to their country's call to service, they now demanded that the nation assure that they not be shunted aside. For wheelchair-bound veterans ... the right to use the same buses and subways as everyone else was, by definition, fundamental.[78]

Groups such as WARPATH (World Association to Remove Prejudice against the Handicapped) used tactics ranging from demonstrations to lobbying and lawsuits.

During the 1960s and early 1970s there were two strands of legal activism on behalf of the growing disability movement. In many states during the 1950s and 1960s the National Federation of the Blind successfully lobbied for the passage of guide dog laws and white cane laws. In addition, a growing number of constitutional challenges were made on behalf of disabled people, particularly mentally handicapped and mentally ill people. Parents of disabled children began to push for a decent education for them. The development of these legal strategies was assisted by the growth of public interest law firms and of rehabilitation and developmental disabilities programmes, which provided funds for the setting up of advocacy projects for people with disabilities.

The growth in militancy and cohesiveness of the disability movement was tremendously boosted by the introduction of a law which for the first time defined disability as a civil rights issue.

The Rehabilitation Act 1973

The first anti-discrimination measure specifically protecting disabled people was passed in 1948, prohibiting discrimination based on physical handicap in United States Civil Service employment. However, since it was never enforced, this measure remained a hollow expression of good will. The Architectural Barriers Act 1968 marked the first federal provision attempting to make the environment more accessible to people with disabilities. It provided for regulations to be devised to establish full accessibility for the disabled public. Grants and loans were to be provided by the government to construct public buildings on condition that they complied with the standards set out in the regulations. The Act followed a report by the National Commission on Architectural Barriers to the Rehabilitation of the Disabled and was supported by the Vocational Rehabilitation Administration on the grounds of cost effectiveness – getting full benefits from rehabilitation services. A prime mover was Hugh Gallagher, a disabled aid to Senator Bartlett.

The earliest attempts to provide civil rights for disabled people sought to amend the Civil Rights Act 1964. Both Representative Charles Vanik and Senator Hubert Humphrey (who had a granddaughter with learning disabilities) introduced such bills in the early 1970s. Both attempts were defeated, probably because civil rights supporters were wary of attempts to extend the scope of the Civil Rights Act beyond what they considered to be the capacity for enforcement.

The breakthrough legislation for disabled civil rights was contained in the Rehabilitation Act, designed to improve the rehabilitation services by shifting from vocational retraining to general independent living programmes. The original draft did not contain any anti-discrimination provisions. These were incorporated during the committee stage and received little legislative attention or indeed publicity. The relevant sections were extremely brief. Section 504 forbade discrimination on the grounds of disability by any programme receiving funding from the federal government; section 501 required the federal government not only to cease discriminating but also to adopt affirmative action programmes for disabled people in its own employment practices; section 503 imposed the same requirements on organisations contracting with the federal government. The potential scope of these provisions was enormous (approximately one-third of the workforce would be covered), but at the time they appear to have been largely understood as a general statement of goodwill. The actual impact of the provisions grew out of the struggles by disabled people to achieve full implementation.

To understand this process it is important first to consider the political context of the period. The most significant factor was the tremendous and inspirational impact of the Civil Rights Movement. This profoundly influenced both the consciousness of those officials whose task it was to implement the law, and the politics of the disability rights groups who struggled to ensure that the full promise of equality contained in the Rehabilitation Act was achieved.

The Rehabilitation Act was passed against the background of the Vietnam war and mass civil unrest. The early 1970s were also a time of heightened tension between a Democratic Congress and the soon to be impeached Republican President Nixon. Many in Congress saw their role as passing sweeping social reforms, to elicit some kind of response from the administration. The means by which such reforms were to be implemented did not receive so much attention.

The Rehabilitation Act was initially vetoed by Nixon because of financial concerns. The first demonstration of disabled people, in 1972, to protest against the veto of the Act was, ironically, that of the President's Committee on the Employment of the Handicapped. They held an all-night vigil at their yearly meeting to honour outstanding disabled people. The following year a further demonstration in support was held.

Drafting the regulations

In 1973, when the Rehabilitation Act was finally passed, Congress had no real grasp of its potential significance. Both the detailed accounts[79] of the development of these sections of the Rehabilitation Act agree that the selection of the agency to formulate the interpreting regulations for the legislation was crucial in determining the ultimate meaning of the Act. The Rehabilitation Services Agency objected to enforcing the sections concerning anti-discrimination. This was fortuitous, since it would presumably have stressed voluntary compliance and community education. The department which was assigned to draft model regulation for all federal agencies was the Office of Civil Rights (OCR) within the Department of Health Education and Welfare (HEW). The OCR had been in the forefront of attempts by the federal government to break racial segregation. Having often faced hostility and prejudice in this effort, it was not organisationally inclined to pursue cooperation, and viewed recipients of federal grants with suspicion. Because there had been so little publicity attached to these sections, the OCR was not subjected to any significant direct interest group pressure during the period when the draft regulations were drawn up. It did however consult disability groups, to use their expertise. After the initial publication of the regulations considerable political pressure did emerge from interest groups representing federal contractors and recipients of federal funds, but there was little subsequent alteration to the regulations. The framework and key concepts were firmly established before these influences brought pressure to bear. Thus disabled activists had a determining influence upon the framework and key concepts of disability anti-discrimination legislation.

Struggle for publication of the regulations

The drafting of the regulations was completed in July 1975; however, intimidated by their potential impact, the government delayed publication. Frustrated by the delays disability groups held further demonstrations. When the Carter administration took over in January 1977 it was initially as cautious as its predecessor. Despite Carter's campaign promise to implement the regulations, he wanted to assess the regulations de novo. Disabled protesters from the ACCD staged sit-ins at the HEW headquarters and regional offices. One official commented: 'We agreed that evicting the blind and the halt and the lame on TV was not quite what the Carter administration needed in its first few months in office.'[80] The administration agreed to issue the regulations forthwith. Demonstrators at Berkeley office remained in occupation until the regulations were actually signed. That occupation lasted 25 days; the regulations were finally signed on 28 April 1977.

Concern about the magnitude of the impact of the regulations could have led them effectively to be buried or have diluted their impact. That this did not happen was the result of advocates in OCR convincing their superiors of the legitimacy of civil rights protection for disabled people and of disabled activists themselves using symbolic gestures to create political, media and popular pressure.

The effect of the government's delay in issuing the regulations was further to politicise the growing disability movement and to make the legislation appear the result of their efforts, rather than a form of bureaucratic paternalism.

The rights-based approach of the Rehabilitation Act was itself a stimulus to the unification of different groups of disabled people. Historically, organisations sought to represent the interests of groups based on a common medical condition – blindness, deafness, cerebral palsy, etc., and these groups then competed against each other for resources from the state. However, once the common experience of discrimination was recognised, this formed the basis for united action. The umbrella organisation, the ACCD, which brought together more than 80 national state and local organisations (such as the American Council for the Blind, National Association of the Deaf, Paralyzed Veterans of America and the National Association for Retarded Citizens) was created in the aftermath of the Rehabilitation Act. Katzman suggests that it is questionable whether the ACCD could have been founded without the rights premise:

> If government defined federal policy towards the disabled as a matter of claims involving the allocation of finite resources, then presumably many of the groups within ACCD would have competed with the others to secure funds for its own constituency. But because the government defined the issue in terms of rights ... each group could champion the demands of the others without financial sacrifice.[81]

The full implementation of the rights recognised in the Rehabilitation Act provided a powerful focus for cohesive action by diverse disability groups, and government resistance merely provoked increased militance.

It would be going too far to say that Section 504 created the disability rights movement of the 1970s, but the existence of Section 504 did strengthen existing national and local organizations and contributed to the development of new ones. The social movement of disabled people became better organized and more broadly based as the result of federal civil rights activities.[82]

Conclusion

This brief consideration of the different processes which have operated historically to exclude disabled people suggests that, since disability is a socially created construct, its meaning can be altered by social and political action. A progressive response will approach disability as a social institution rather than a medical problem; it must seek to counter the legacy and lingering dominance of segregation and exclusion, and to overturn a model of provision which is dominated by the control of professionals and the enforced dependency of disabled people.

The history of discrimination, and the evidence of continuing discrimination, provide a powerful moral justification for incurring significant social costs, if necessary, in order to remedy the effects of past discrimination, and by so doing to shape a society that is more inclusive of the full range of abilities within it.

The American history of contrasting provision points the way to an alternative legislative response to disability. The full impact of such a model is explored in Chapters 3 and 4. First, however, Chapter 2 seeks to provide a theoretical basis for this examination by considering critiques of the use of a rights discourse as a route to social equality.

2
Law's Power over Inequality

This chapter examines law's potential to act as a positive agent of social change, specifically the extent to which creating a legal right to equal and non-discriminatory treatment advances the position of disadvantaged groups. It considers critiques of a rights-based approach, framed in relation to sex and race legislation, and looks at their relevance to the position of disabled people, in particular the suggestion that disability as a basis for categorisation is so fundamentally different from race or gender that it is inappropriate to use the same rights-based framework.

In so far as the criticisms of rights legislation relate to the gap between ideal and reality, to operational weaknesses such as questions of access, implementation and enforcement, these crucial issues will be a continuing theme, discussed at various points in the book. This chapter concentrates on the arguments that the failure of rights legislation stems from a flawed ideal. In a sense this is an artificial distinction, the problems of implementation not being separate from but integral to the theoretical critiques of the form of legislation, but it is easier to understand the barriers to implementation once we have addressed the underlying theoretical issues.

It is helpful to start with a broad consideration of the nature of law, its power and limitations.

The complicity of law

> [I]f law cannot deliver on its promise to transcend power, it must conceal power, and the power of the law is, therefore, in large measure ideological, that is to say it makes social relations based on power appear legitimate and just because they appear to be beyond power.[1]

One of the distinctive characteristics of law as a social institution is its claim to impartiality. Law's claim to be apart from and above politics, economics and culture, to offer an objective, quasi-scientific analysis which results in 'fairness' and 'justice', is key to its legitimacy and symbolic power. Even where judges are accused of bias, or judgements are described as 'fixed', these are presented as departures from an idealised model of neutral judicial decision-making.

A critique of these pretensions to impartiality is the essential starting point for any radical assessment of law's powers and limitations. Both feminists and anti-racists have asserted the partiality of legal discourse, not only despite but because of its claims to universality and rationality. The law has historically only been capable of putting forward its partial viewpoint as a universalist one by discounting whole categories of persons – women, slaves, aliens, and disabled people who have been labelled as 'incompetents'.

Fitzpatrick relates law's claims to universality to the racist legacy of the Enlightenment, whose 'terrifying consistency puts the enslaved and the colonised beyond the liberal equation of universal freedom and equality by rendering them in racist terms as qualitatively different.'[2] The potential contradiction between law's claims to universality and its confinement to a specific national community is likewise resolved by portraying law as an expression of national superiority, 'the incarnation of a rational universal ordering'. Fitzpatrick traces this legacy even within the race relations law, the purported aim of which is to stop discrimination. He quotes the then Home Secretary, William Whitelaw, who pronounced that the price of such protection was that these 'ethnic minorities' should 'demonstrate their commitment to our society', and abandon 'cultural and linguistic isolation'.[3]

Feminists too have refuted the neutrality of law, arguing that the structure of its discourse is inherently partial and privileges the male. Gilligan, for example, critiques the impersonal, objective and unemotional ideology of Western jurisprudence, counterposing to it a feminine model which is caring and situational.[4] In a similar vein Smart describes law as 'phallogocentric', a combination of

> phallocentric, which is the masculine heterosexual imperative, and logocentric, which is the term appropriated by feminists to identify the fact that knowledge is not neutral but produced under conditions of patriarchy ... The constitution of law and the constitution of masculinity may overlap and share mutual resonances.[5]

She distinguishes her argument from Gilligan's psycho-biological determinism by inviting readers to consider the developments of the professions of nursing and the law and recognise the way in which the discourses which constitute these professions are intrinsically overlaid by the discourses of femininity and masculinity.

The limits of law

These critiques illustrate the importance of refusing to reify 'The Law'. That is to say, the law must not be regarded as a social force in its own right, but rather the product of specific interests, which can only take effect through a variety of social institutions (of which legal institutions form a crucial strand, but not the entirety), within which a variety of competing influences operate to determine the outcome:

> Thus, when we ask whether law can promote social change, we are really considering whether the actions of those members of the population who ... have been able to get their demands of interests recognised by law will be successful in overcoming resistance to the pursuance through law of their claims. Law is not, therefore, an actor in itself but only the instrument of the human actors whose interests it represents.[6]

This makes the analysis of law's effectiveness much more complex. The specific impact of discrete legislative measures must be placed within a broader understanding of the forces that produced them, and that influence their implementation.

In this light, I would argue that those critics who contrast the failure of legal measures with the necessity for political commitment are mistaken in counterposing these as alternative strategies. Thus, Lustgarten and Edwards contend that institutional discrimination and social disadvantage require more subtle long-term policies, capable of adaptation in the light of chance and experience, and that rights must be subordinated to a policy-orientated approach. Ideally they propose that every policy decision should be vetted in advance for its impact – decisions such as the location of key industries or the level of construction of public sector housing. They compare reliance upon legal tools with 'trying to etch figures in glass with a pick axe'.[7] But this juxtaposition of laws and political policy is misplaced, since laws are frequently the essential instruments of policy and politicians, however unwieldy they may prove for the degree of precision engineering which is required.

Undoubtedly broader policy changes can produce more immediately powerful effects, but this assumes a pre-existing level of political commitment. Rights laws can themselves be used as part of a broader campaign to produce the leverage required to increase such political commitment, as indeed happened with American disability legislation. In contrast, Lustgarten and Edwards' proposed mechanism for ensuring the required political commitment is transparently weak – a cabinet committee chaired by a senior minister.

Equally, it is important not to ask too much of individual pieces of legislation, by abstracting them from the surrounding context of broader social and economic changes. The Civil Rights Act 1964, for example, did produce a marked improvement in the labour market position of black workers, but failed to prevent a massive increase in black poverty. One of the most significant reasons for this development was changes in the labour market which produced huge unemployment in precisely those areas and those occupations in which blacks had traditionally predominated. This is not to say that such a development was unrelated to the prevalence of institutional racism, but to point out the need to look at the broader picture to provide a realistic measure of the effectiveness of rights legislation.

Such laws cannot be expected to substitute for a broader politics, capable of addressing the wider policy issues and of providing the push required to operationalise legislation. It is necessary to understand the extent to which rights legislation can provide a useful tool and weapon for such a broader political struggle, and which areas are more amenable to a rights strategy than others. For example, where demands are placed on the state's resources, any 'rights' will inevitably be constrained by its concern to maintain control of the process by which these are rationed. Nevertheless, even in these areas the existence of a broader rights-based framework can both prove a potent weapon for demanding more resources, and powerfully influence the context in which resources are delivered. (This issue is discussed in the disability context in Chapter 7.)

The power of law

A further lesson of anti-racist and feminist critiques of law is the important role which it plays in forming the ideological system which is hegemonic within society, legitimating a specific set of values and assumptions. The law provides the framework within which groups and individuals interpret the nature of their interests and the conflicts with other groups. Precisely because of law's power to define, it is acknowledged to be an important site of struggle and resource for groups seeking social change. Smart describes it as a 'forum for articulating alternative visions and accounts.'[8]

This symbolic function suggests that the effectiveness of law does not purely depend on whether it can be invoked or enforced. I will argue later that the inclusion of disability within an equal rights rather than a welfare framework marks a tremendous leap forward ideologically. First, however, it is necessary to consider the negative aspects of the message of rights discourse.

Law individualises

Marxists and critical legal theorists identify the individualism of law within capitalist countries as its most distinctive characteristic. The seminal account is that of Pashunakis, who argues that law under capitalism characteristically regards the rights and duties of all individuals as equal before the law which it claims to be impartial, and by so doing disguises the real structures of inequality.[9] Cotterell characterises legal individualism thus:

> The individualism embodied in modern law stresses above all that individuals are makers of their own destiny; standing alone they bear responsibility for the acts and omissions attributed to them ... Thus, in its purest form, it takes no account of social or cultural factors that may remove the possibility of choice from individual actors, or severely limit the choices available to them, or determine the way these choices are interpreted.[10]

An important strand of criticism of rights-based strategies is that by reducing people to isolated individuals they run counter to the only possible basis for such progress, which is collective action. Whilst it is true that legal action can channel individuals' energies in this way, I believe that this depends fundamentally on the broader context within which the law is operationalised. I will argue that the American experience with civil rights, particularly for disabled people, contradicts this account by providing examples of the power of rights-based ideology and activity to forge a collective identity.

From a feminist and anti-racist perspective, theorists have criticised the extent to which the dominant legal model of equality operates on a classically individualised basis, which fails to address the deep structural inequalities within our society. Equality is understood within this paradigm as meaning the right to be treated in the same way and given the same opportunities as those who already have them. Thus, for example, the British Race Relations Act 1976 states that a person discriminates against another if 'on racial grounds he treats that other less favourably than he treats or would treat other persons'.[11] The definition of discrimination in the Sex Discrimination Act 1975 is identically framed.

Perhaps the most glaring evidence that these laws (and the comparable American provisions in the Civil Rights Act 1964) have been framed in a way which ignores structural inequalities is the way in which they extend equal protection to advantaged and disadvantaged groups. White men are deemed by the form of these laws to require as much protection from discrimination as black women. This 'even-handedness' is a powerful feature of the sex and race laws, and has been particularly important in constraining the extent to which positive action can be taken to compensate for the past discrimination experienced by women and black people.

This model, the formal equality model, is premised upon the existence of a neutrally functioning, non-discriminatory society where only isolated acts of irrational discrimination occur. It is cast in a negative fashion, prohibiting actions which can be shown to be discriminatory, and thus focuses upon discrete, individual acts of discrimination, and in particular upon the issue of motivation.

This analysis applies the tort framework to anti-discrimination law, so that an employer will only incur liability if s/he is personally responsible for the harm suffered by an individual. This responsibility is understood in terms of a simplified model of causation which does not include responsibility for the effects of failure to act, and in particular does not recognise liability for failure to correct the impact of past discrimination. Conaghan and Mansell in their critique of tort law discuss how this assessment of omissions as incurring less liability than acts reflects the economic and political perspective of market capitalism.[12] They argue that capitalism opposes the imposition of positive obligations on people on the basis that it constrains capitalist freedom and hence limits economic growth. We will see that a desire to cater to the needs of business and to limit costs has indeed been a powerful constraint on the operation of anti-discrimination laws.

Charles Lawrence describes the consequence of this model as the law's complete inability to address the deep structural inequalities faced by Afro-Americans:

> the existing intent requirement's assignment of individualized fault or responsibility for the existence of racial discrimination distorts our perceptions about the causes of discrimination and leads us to think about racism in a way that advances the disease rather than combatting it. By insisting that a blameworthy perpetrator be found before the existence of racial discrimination can be acknowledged, the Court creates an imaginary world where discrimination does not exist unless intended. By acting as if this imaginary world was real and insisting that we participate in this fantasy, the Court and the law it promulgates subtly shape our perceptions of society ... if blacks are being fairly treated yet remain at the bottom of the socio-economic ladder, only their own inferiority can explain their subordinate position.[13]

I agree that the formal equality model is fundamentally flawed because it does not recognise, or seek to redress, structural inequalities. Furthermore, because it fails to do so this model cannot succeed in redressing inequality, and risks compounding the problem by legitimating inequality through its false account of equality.

The formal equality model described above is the dominant jurisprudential model for equality legislation (including constitutional protection) in both Britain and America. However, there are other strands within equality laws which are more capable of achieving positive change, because they reflect a more realistic understanding of the operation of discrimination. We will examine these within the context of their ability to respond to the issue of difference.

Difference

Because the formal model of equality requires that similarly situated people be treated in a similar fashion it can only operate in the absence of any relevant differences between members of protected groups and the rest of the workforce. For women, as for black and disabled people, assertions by the dominant groups that they are different have invariably meant less valued, carrying a tremendous stigma, even when disguised as compliments about nurturing natures or moral purity. This creates an enormous pressure to deny the presence of significant differences, and initially feminists concentrated on critiquing assertions of gender differences, exposing myths or stereotypes such as that women were less good at science or as leaders. This strategy was consistent with the understanding of discrimination in the formal equality model as either animosity towards, or the use of stereotypes about, certain groups.

Undoubtedly this initial work is essential if women are to break into previously exclusive, male areas of society. In addition, the formal equality model can also protect the non-average members of a class, by scrutinising inaccurate generalisations. For example, if employers require employees of a certain minimum height, they will not be entitled to exclude women as a class on the basis that the average woman will not meet the height specification, but must assess applicants individually. However, the limitations of this assimilationist imperative quickly became apparent. In recent years many feminist theorists have highlighted the centrality of genuine differences between the sexes in preventing women from achieving equality, and the consequent inadequacy of the formal equality model. Scales, for example, asserts: 'The relevant differences have been, and always will be those which keep women in their place.'[14] Dickens comments:

> There is a song in the musical *My Fair Lady* which asks 'Why Can't a Woman be more Like a Man?' This might be the theme tune for the world of paid work. The more a woman is like a man ... the better she will fare in employment ... The more she differs from this male norm, through having an interrupted or irregular employment pattern, or through combining primary care responsibilities with paid work, then the ... greater the disadvantages she will experience.[15]

For disadvantaged groups these differences from the white, male, able-bodied 'norm' are often clearly the historical legacy of discriminatory treatment.

Racial disadvantage in the fullest sense is outside the law entirely. By racial disadvantage we mean material, psychological or social inequalities, bearing disproportionately upon racial minorities. Examples are under achievement in schooling, higher rates of unemployment or residential concentration in decaying neighbourhoods. Discrimination is both a major element and a continuing long-term cause of disadvantage, but the latter has a self-perpetuating dynamic of its own.[16]

For example, one common legacy of historical exclusion from a workplace is that black or female workers have less seniority within a firm than its 'traditional' workforce. Therefore operating a mode of selection for redundancy which appears to be fair, because it treats everyone in the same way, can actually be grossly unfair since it perpetuates the effects of past discrimination. The classic 'last in first out' formula would inevitably mean that more black and female workers were made redundant. Similarly, discrimination outside the workplace can mean that different groups do not come to work on equal terms. In the landmark Supreme Court case of Griggs (discussed on pp.39–40 below) broader societal discrimination meant that black applicants were less likely to have the high school diplomas which a firm was requiring of employees. Because this level of qualification bore no relevance to the jobs in question it was argued that this criteria was unfair.

The formal equality model is incapable of addressing these types of discrimination, because it ignores the broader structural differences between groups, and reifies these disadvantaged social positions into differences between individuals.

One of the key historical legacies for women is occupational segregation by gender, which remains very powerful. An American study in 1980 estimated that 57 per cent of women would have had to change their occupation in order for them to have had the same occupational distribution as men.[17] Another American study estimated that nearly four-fifths of the wage gap between the sexes can be attributed to the different distributions of women and men across occupations.[18] In Britain the same pattern exists. A TUC report, *Women in the Labour Market*,[19] found women concentrated in a small number of industries and predominantly in a handful of occupations – shop work, clerical, secretarial, catering, cleaning and routine assembly line jobs. Women represented only 0.8 per cent of the Institute of Mechanical Engineers,[20] and the 'glass ceiling' means there are still few women at the top of professions, industry or commerce. In 1991 only 11 per cent of women were in professional or managerial positions, whilst women constituted only 4 per cent of senior and middle management positions, and 1–2 per cent of senior executives.

The huge extent of occupational segregation inevitably means that many jobs become structured to suit the needs of one particular gender. Dickens describes as the 'key to women's disadvantage in the labour market' the fact that the 'structures of employment, although apparently neutral, are in fact moulded around the life patterns and domestic obligations of men.'[21] Her account contrasts the full-time, regular, permanent work on the employer's premises of the standard male worker with the part-time, temporary working and homeworking of many women.

This gendered structure can be subtle but pervasive. I have already quoted Smart's comments on the masculine nature of the legal profession, contrasted with the 'feminine' mould of the nursing profession; other studies address a range of professions.[22]

One of the most powerful forms which discrimination takes both for women and for people from ethnic minorities is the simple feeling that they 'do not fit in'. Their potential contribution to a workplace is devalued because they do not measure up to the conventional way in which the job has been performed or because they are seen as causing disruption in the workplace. The case of *Singh* v. *The Chief Constable of the Nottingham Constabulary CID* questioned the police's unacknowledged standard that people should behave and be exactly like those already in CID, despite the fact that there might be equally effective ways of doing the job.[23]

The legacy of exclusion from occupations can take more concrete forms. Sexual and racial harassment as a response to the intrusion of new workers into a previously homogenous workforce is a very powerful barrier to the full integration of workplaces. Fifty-four per cent of women interviewed in a survey by the Industrial Society were the victims of sexual harassment.[24] This factor imposed a very real cost for both the individuals involved and the employing organisations, in terms of the impact on their work. Harassment was found to result in an inability to concentrate, loss of confidence, etc. An even more powerful legacy is the lack of flexibility in 'male' occupations required to take into account historical gender roles – such as women's primary responsibility for childcare and the 'double shift' of domestic labour. Part-time work is almost invariably female work – 87 per cent of part-time workers are women.[25] Career patterns in many jobs are as inflexible as working patterns. A career break to have children is frequently fatal for a high flier.

These deeply embedded patterns in the 'private sphere' have a powerful impact upon women's employment opportunities – confining women to jobs which are compatible with their 'family responsibilities'. Occupations which have become labelled as 'female' tend to take on a structure which is compatible with women's role in the home, while 'male' occupations tend to have a structure which conflicts with that role.

It is no accident that many of these areas of difference from the white male 'norm' stem from areas ruled out by law. Smart talks of the limits beyond which the law will not proceed, of confining categories constituting the domain of the normal.[26] By not entering areas where sexism and racism are prevalent, the law implicitly confers power on those who are dominant within them. Attacks on single mothers both in Britain and America have greatly increased the proportion of the female workforce which is trapped in poverty – undercutting the progress generated by the equality laws and in some case forcing them out of the regular workforce as they become reliant on welfare and the 'black market economy'. At the other end of the social spectrum the 1993 'Nannygate' fiasco, in which successive female appointees to the position of US Attorney-General were revealed to have employed illegal immigrant women as childminders, was a vivid reminder of the pervasive impact of the lack of state childcare provision.

Even where distinctions between the sexes, such as pregnancy, are physiological these 'real' differences take their meaning from the social context in which they are manifested. A simple example is the fact that often the equipment in a 'male' occupation is not suited to the height or build of the average female.[27] This can either be explained as a result of biological differences, as it would be in the formal equality analysis, or it can be understood as the result of the structural exclusion of women from these occupations.

I have dwelt at some length on the centrality of 'difference' in the marginalisation of all discriminated against groups, and the parallels with the situation of disabled people becomes obvious in this last example. We will see in the next chapter the argument that disabled people are different from able-bodied people has been put forward by many commentators as distinguishing them from other 'minority' groups. As the above discussion makes clear, this problem of difference is a shared experience of these different 'minorities', and I will now consider some proposed mechanisms for taking it into account within equality discourse.

Special treatment – reasonable accommodation

One response to the issue of differences is to ignore them and continue to promote formal equality for the minority that can benefit. In America the issue crystallised for women over the question of whether to pursue an Equal Rights Amendment (ERA) to the Constitution, which would grant women more equality, but at the expense of extending the sway of the formal equality model. Gregory comments that the proponents of the ERA believed that 'the only way to undermine the sexual division of labour was to ignore it'.[28] A contrasting response is to leave the basic structure of the workplace untouched, but provide special treatment to address those needs of protected groups which are additional to those of the 'normal' workforce members.

There is a long history of special treatment for women, in the form of protective legislation. Historically these laws were not framed within the context of equality. And this history raises suspicions of the incompatibility of special treatment with equality, that rather than complementing formal equality it undermines it. In the words of one critic: 'Any permitted difference in treatment as between men and women is likely to protect away women's liberties.'[29]

The debate has tended to focus particularly around pregnancy, and this itself is an indication of the narrow reach of special treatment, which does not seek to grapple with the broader differences. Still it is interesting to look at the debate in some detail, because the special treatment approach is precisely the one which the American legislation has employed to deal with the physical or mental differences of disability.

Krieger and Cooney argue that equality for women requires special treatment to take into account real sexual differences, and they give the example of the importance of employers providing adequate maternity leave.[30] These American proponents of the special treatment approach suggest the adoption and expansion of the reasonable accommodation approach, which originated in Civil Rights Act case law relating to religious discrimination, as a means of complementing the formal equality analysis. This requires that employers make reasonable efforts to structure work schedules in order to accommodate employees' religious observances.

However, this approach carries with it two fundamental problems. On a practical level, because it accepts the existing structure as a given, this will inevitably place severe limitations on the extent of alterations which courts will be prepared to order. On an ideological level, this approach perpetuates the stigmatisation of difference. Catharine MacKinnon criticises both the traditional equal treatment doctrine and the use of the special treatment approach to supplement it on this basis, arguing that in effect they give women a choice of being either like men with equal treatment, or different from men with 'special treatment'.[31]

Taub and Williams similarly describe the proposal of special accommodation for women as a very dangerous concept which treats equality as a form of noblesse oblige:

> It presents itself as a question of how far employers will be required to deviate from 'standard' procedures, laid down for their 'normal' employees, in order to take into account the special problems of abnormal workers. Not surprisingly courts will not carry such an idea

very far, and, also not surprisingly, 'accommodation' labels the workers to whom accommodation is made as 'different' ... and in a large part, a burden.[32]

Martha McCluskey argues, in the context of disability discrimination, that terming the needs of people with disabilities 'special' continues to accept the able-bodied person as the norm:

> This view fails to recognize that disability is normal. The needs of people with disabilities such as the need for ramps instead of stairs are basic human needs shared by large numbers of people. All people have physical limitations and all can expect to have more disabilities as they grow older.[33]

By taking able-bodied people as the norm this view continues to locate the 'problem' in the physical/mental impairments of disabled people, rather than in a society which has been organised to exclude them. Just as a society which was not designed to exclude women would have workplace policies and social structures that would prevent pregnancy from impairing women's careers, so a society designed to include people of all abilities would design buses with ramps and low floors.

McCluskey urges that the able-bodied norm needs to be replaced by a standard which embodies the full range of human experience. She points out that there are other important social needs which employers are expected to meet, such as vacation time, but that historically only those needs which have been associated with the able-bodied, male work norm have been taken into account.

The disparate impact model
These critiques point to the stigmatising effect of the formal equality and special treatment approaches, arguing that the structural dominance of the white, able-bodied norm causes difference to become equated with stigma in our society. To counter the equation of difference with stigma, we need to focus not on similarities and differences but on the conditions that produce these, and thereby challenge the power that is attached to the labelling and the construction of hierarchies of difference. Finley argues with regard to sex discrimination,[34] and McCluskey with respect to disability discrimination,[35] that the disparate impact doctrine (and its British equivalent, 'indirect discrimination') provides a legal mechanism for analysing, in precisely this way, the social conditions which produce difference.

Judicial interpretation of the Civil Rights Act in America developed two different doctrinal models. The first of these, the disparate treatment model, focuses on the intent of the employer, and as such falls squarely into the formal equality analysis. However, in the ground-breaking case of *Griggs* v. *Duke Power Co.*[36] the Supreme Court recognised the inability of a law which focuses on the motives of individuals to challenge long-standing discriminatory practices, and devised a new doctrinal model which examines consequences rather than intentions. In this case the Court interpreted the Civil Rights Act as also prohibiting employment practices, regardless of the employer's intent, where they have a discriminatory effect on protected classes, unless the employer can justify them as being required by business necessity. This is known as the disparate impact doctrine:

> Congress has now provided that tests or criteria for employment ... may not provide equality of opportunity merely in the sense of the fabled offer of milk to the stork and the fox. On the contrary Congress has now required that the posture and condition of the job-seeker be taken into account. It has – to resort again to the fable – provided that the vessel in which the milk is proffered be one all seekers can use. The Act proscribes not only overt discrimination but also practices that are fair in form, but discriminatory in operation.[37]

This quotation is suggestive of the ideological and practical potential of this approach, in that it can address a model of discrimination which is structural. The potency of indirect discrimination lies in the fact that it goes beyond the realm of the individual, conceptualising discrimination as involving more than episodic wrongdoing. The principle of scrutinising practices for disparate impact exposes the white, able-bodied male frame of reference and fosters a collective understanding that an employer's use of exclusionary 'neutral' practices is both unfair and counter-productive from a social perspective.

In practice, the courts have been unwilling to adopt such a radical interpretation of the disparate impact doctrine. The justification given in the Griggs case itself for the disparate impact investigation is that it is necessary to stop the perpetuation of past discrimination and that 'the national interest in eliminating employment discrimination overrides the employer's interest in administrative convenience and cost saving'.[38] However, the Griggs opinion also stated that 'The touchstone is business necessity.'[39] The issue on which litigation has thus focused is how to interpret 'business necessity', how much weight to give the competing factors of cost saving to the employer and remedying the social evil of discrimination. Generally courts have largely focused on the issue of whether practices are productive in terms of the business in question, rather than on considering the social perspective.[40] This reluctance to impose upon individual employers the cost of restructuring their businesses to take account of broader historical and social factors is a limitation contained within all anti-discrimination jurisprudence.[41]

The narrower holding in Griggs was that selection criteria should be functionally relevant and measure the applicant's ability to perform rather than measuring abstract qualities or functionally extraneous characteristics. If neutral requirements have a disparate impact on protected groups they will be presumed to be invalid unless they can be justified by the employer as being related to job performance. In practical terms the shifting of the burden of persuasion on to the employer has been an invaluable tool for pushing American employers to move towards more integrated workplaces.

Thus, although this doctrine has been given a broader interpretation by some theorists, it is primarily an extension of the requirement that businesses should be operated in a rational way. This dominant interpretation of the disparate impact doctrine therefore still fits within the formal equality model – since it relies on the absence of any *relevant* differences between a member of a protected group and the white, Christian, able-bodied norm. As such it leaves untouched the effects of historical and structural exclusion, measuring the efficiency of practices in terms of the existing structure of the workplace.

British legislation

The British anti-discrimination legislation prohibits direct discrimination where an individual is less favourably treated than a person of the opposite sex or another racial group would have been treated. Although there is no requirement in either the Race Relations Act 1976 or the Sex Discrimination Act 1975 that the employer should have intended to discriminate, in most cases the motives of the employer are the central issue.

The additional concept of indirect discrimination was included because of a visit to the US by Roy Jenkins (at that time Home Secretary). A person is said indirectly to discriminate under the Race Relations Act if

he applies to that other a requirement or condition which he applies or would apply equally to persons not of the same racial group as that other but:

i) which is such that the proportion of persons of the same racial groups as that other who can comply with it is considerably smaller than the proportion of persons not of that racial group who can comply with it; and

ii) which he cannot show to be justifiable irrespective of the colour, nationality or ethnic origins of the person to whom it is applied; and

iii) which is to the detriment of that other because he cannot comply with it.[42]

The Sex Discrimination Act contains an identical provision against indirect discrimination.[43]

In Britain, however, the potency of indirect discrimination has been blunted far more than it has in America by judicial decisions which give a very broad interpretation of whether or not a condition is 'justifiable'.

I will consider the reasons for this relative failure in Britain in more detail in Chapter 6.

Positive action

The Commission for Racial Equality (CRE) argues that any system which aims to achieve racial equality must recognise the mode of operation of racial discrimination, in particular that it is not practised openly and that 'much of it is perpetrated by people who are unaware that they are racially discriminating'.[44] The concept of indirect discrimination, it suggests, can help tackle these features:

> The only way in which the presence of racial discrimination, including covert and unintentional acts, can be routinely revealed is the ethnic monitoring of the relevant decisions. The whole experience of the Commission points to this central conclusion. No organisation can be sure that racial discrimination is not occurring unless it has such a system in place.[45]

Furthermore, where such discrimination is revealed, action should be taken to remedy it.

The broader social and historical disadvantages suffered by certain groups mean that laws which merely impose minimal standards are not sufficient to promote anything like equality in practical terms. That is, they might result in equal treatment but will not produce any significant change in outcomes, or in the position of disadvantaged groups. Aggressive good practice aiming at results is required to produce change. Affirmative action is the term by which such proactive attempts to alter the composition of the workforce is known. Although the term has become associated in the popular consciousness with 'quotas' – fixed proportions of the workforce which employers seek to fill with members of disadvantaged groups – it is in fact a far more subtle concept. Affirmative action is certainly a far more complex attempt to address the problem of difference than the 'special treatment/reasonable accommodation' approach considered above, although such measures may be incorporated into a programme.

The CRE carefully distinguishes 'equality targets' from quotas:

We do not advocate quotas, under which set percentages of a workforce would be reserved for particular ethnic groups ... Equality targets can be established on the basis of what might be expected to happen in the absence of decision-making on racial grounds ... If targets are not met, then searching out the reasons may help reveal the incidence of racial discrimination ... which can then be tackled.[46]

Affirmative action involves analysing the barriers which have resulted in the disproportionate employment of white, able-bodied men, and seeking to overcome those barriers by a variety of means. Thus, it might typically involve outreach recruitment targeted at particularly under-represented groups, remedial training for groups who have less access to the normal training channels, as well as measures such as childcare provision which address the differing needs outside the workplace.

Monitoring the present proportion of disadvantaged groups within the various sections of the workforce is an essential part of this process, as it provides an indication of the problem to be resolved. Similarly, many organisations believe that drawing up targets to provide a measure of the success of affirmative action policies is an equally essential component of any effective positive action policy.

In the sense that such policies necessitate focusing on the differences between disadvantaged groups and the white, able-bodied male 'norm', and treating groups differently on the basis of the very characteristics which the formal equality model insists should be ignored (sex, race, religion or disability), such policies contrast sharply with the formal equality model. It is crucial that the justification for this 'preferential' treatment is understood. As Meehan puts it: 'it is important to resist the charge that affirmative or positive action means treating protected groups more favourably and to remind opponents that it compensates for past discrimination and widens the pool of qualified applicants'.[47] One of the Supreme Court cases which drew up the boundaries of acceptable positive action in America succinctly describes the reason why positive action is needed: 'Congress did not intend to freeze an entire generation of Negro employees into discriminatory patterns that existed before the Act'.[48]

American, but (as we will see in Chapter 6) not British courts have the power to order positive action programmes as a remedy where discriminatory practices have been proved. This power was frequently used in the 1970s. In addition, affirmative action programmes were frequently adopted voluntarily by employers in order to fend off potential suits under Title VII of the Civil Rights Act. Such cases, particularly where class actions were involved, would entail damaging publicity and potentially huge costs.[49]

Affirmative action falls within the substantive equality paradigm rather than the formal equality model. It moves the rights approach away from the individualism which, we have seen, crucially restricts its operation:

Reducing segregation involves widespread general changes and solutions that affect whole firms and industries. American legal procedures and legally imposed affirmative action policies go a long way towards adapting a legal system that is based on individual rights, remedies and sanctions into a suitable vehicle for solving collective problems.[50]

The potency of rights discourse

Because it is logically incoherent and manipulable ... rights discourse is a trap ... one is without guidance in deciding what to do about fundamental questions and fated to the gradual loss of confidence in the convincingness of what one has to say ... Liberal rights analysis submerges the student in legal rhetoric but because of its inherent vacuousness, can provide no more than an emotional stance against the legal order![51]

Carol Smart, despite her broader critiques of feminists' tendency to legal solutions, recognises that this 'emotional stance' is precisely one of the great strengths of rights discourse. 'To couch a claim in terms of rights is a major step towards a recognition of a social wrong ... It is also the case that to pose an issue in terms of rights is to make the claim "popular"'[52] (by which she means accessible to popular debate). Regardless of any inherent philosophical incoherence, this is a powerful resource.

Having analysed some of the limitations of the anti-discrimination framework, I want to stress its value. Basing disabled people's claims on a rights discourse has practical political advantages:

Characterizing access as a civil right had distinct political advantages. To portray access as another government benefit ... would have defined improved access as desirable but not a social imperative. Allowing disabled people greater participation thus would become an essentially charitable act. In periods of limited resources ... it is politically acceptable to limit benevolent acts of charity ... Reducing benefits may be legitimate, while violating rights is not.[53]

However, this model's ideological significance is even more important: a rights-based discourse has a great capacity for empowering disabled people and for beneficially shaping broader social discourse. Even whilst Carol Smart warns that rights do not resolve problems, she accepts their value in transposing the problem into one which is defined as having a legal solution.[54] As long as the exclusion, segregation and second-class treatment of disabled people is seen as their individual problem, caused by their physical or mental impairment, the solution will continue to be posed in terms of a medical cure or charitable dependency. To recast it in terms of structural discrimination is to present the solution in terms of changes to society:

> For the historically disempowered, the conferring of rights is symbolic of all the denied aspects of humanity: rights imply a respect which places one within the referential range of self and others, which elevates one's status from human body to human being.[55]

Written from a black perspective, these words apply with equal force to disabled people, who have for so long had their humanity denied, and been deprived of the capacity for self-determination. The very articulation of a right to equal, non-segregated access to social institutions has had a tremendous force both for shaping broader public discourse and for the individual and collective empowerment of disabled people.

Just as 'the locus of women's subordination is frequently the private and individual sphere ... and is thus ... experienced in isolation',[56] so the subordination of disabled people has been located by society in the incapacities of their own bodies. Casting access requirements in the framework of rights discourse locates disabled people's subordination in the public rather than the private sphere. It therefore promotes a sense of collective identity amongst disabled people who, despite the vast differences in their individual disabilities, share a common experience of exclusion and stigmatisation by society.

Rights discourses can help form the self-definition of disabled people as well as their collective identity. Because of the historical stigma attached to the word 'disabled' (or, still more, 'handicapped') many have denied this label. President Roosevelt would not have considered himself 'handicapped' – and indeed went to great lengths to conceal the effects of polio. However, as a wheelchair user, he undoubtedly experienced difficulties created by society's exclusion of people with mobility impairments. As disability comes to be understood as a form of discrimination, rather than as a personal failing, and as the stigma attached to the label becomes weaker, more people will be prepared to accept this identity.

Ironically, this contradicts the common argument that because law reduces people to isolated individuals it runs counter to the only possible basis for radical change – collective action. Rights discourse promotes the development of an individual's sense of self and a group's collective identity most powerfully through the process in which these rights are asserted. The act of claiming a right is itself an assertion of moral self-worth. The advocacy process itself, for a group like disabled people who have historically been excluded from public life, combats this exclusion. Through the process of political action disabled people consolidate their sense of group identity and pride and, by requiring the development of political and organisational skills, disabled people are enabled to acquire political power.

Thus, the growth of the American disability movement was the result of an increase in self- and collective-identification of disabled people, while this increase was itself, in part, produced by the collective efforts to assert and enforce the right of equal opportunity contained, embryonically, in the Rehabilitation Act 1973.

Schneider argues that the power of rights discourse lies in the 'dynamic interrelationship of rights and politics'. In the context of the women's movement she explores:

> [The] way in which the assertion of 'experience' of rights can express political vision, affirm a group's humanity, contribute to an individual's development as a whole person, and assist in the collective political development of a social or political movement, particularly in its early stages.[57]

The history of the Rehabilitation Act and Americans with Disabilities Act is powerful testimony to the aptness of this description with regards to the disability movement.

It is a paradox, in no way unique to disabled people, that the anti-discrimination approach requires that in order to assert their right to full and equal participation in society, they must continue to assert their differences. The price of being heard, and achieving some control over the consequences of disability, is to accept the label. The power of the argument that disability is social myth, constructed out of the range of physical and mental limitations which are the inevitable consequences of being human, is lost. Liggett describes this limitation: 'The minority group approach is double-edged because it means enlarging the discursive practices which participate in the constitution of disability. The new perspectives then become involved in disciplining disability.'[58]

Perhaps the situation is most similar to that of lesbians and gay men. A radical approach to sexuality understands it, in Freud's famous phrase, as 'polymorphously perverse', involving a spectrum of shifting objects of desire, which becomes understood as 'heterosexual' and 'homosexual' as the result of historical social processes unique to Western late capitalism.[59] The act of proclaiming 'a lesbian identity' or 'gay rights' undercuts this understanding. However, for the individual humans who are the bearers of these social constructions the power of the assertion of a common identity, and of claiming protection as a minority group, cannot be overestimated.

Part of the power of invoking a gay or lesbian identity is its ability through the assertion of a collective 'gay pride' to reverse the assumptions and cure the wounds inflicted on an individual by a homophobic society. Similarly, an important aspect of the assertion of a common disabled identity is its extension beyond the shared experience of oppression, to a positive evaluation of 'disability culture'. The deaf community and the disability arts movement are the most developed examples of this aspect of the disability movement.

Recognising the power of rights discourse is not to deny the importance of retaining non-legal strategies, to 'de-centre' law. Smart stresses the importance of resisting the 'temptation which law offers, namely the promise of a solution'.[60] She offers a complex view of law's power, one that is 'refracted' so that it is not possible to develop a grand theory or strategy about its usefulness as a source of social reform. She acknowledges the value of the first-generation feminist law reforms, whilst questioning the value of extending rights discourse into new areas. I would argue that the assertion of disability rights is comparable to the first wave of feminist or black civil rights, a powerful reformulation of problems which had previously been individualised and pathologised into social problems.

Is disability discrimination different?

Chapter 3 examines the American anti-discrimination legislation for people with disabilities in the light of the above critiques. However, a preliminary question which presents itself is whether disability is capable of being addressed within the same framework as sex and race.

The level of resistance from the courts to the concept that disabled people experience discrimination is exemplified in the Supreme Court case of *City of Cleburne* v. *Cleburne Living Center*,[61] which denies mentally handicapped people any but the most basic level of scrutiny under the equal protection clause of the constitution.

The evaluation that the judgement places on this disability is clear from the footnote which quotes Dean Ely: 'Surely one has to feel sorry for a person disabled by something he or she can't do anything about, but I'm not aware of any reason to suppose that elected officials are unlikely to share that feeling.'[62] While the judgement acknowledges that 'there have been and there will continue to be instances of discrimination' it is clear that the Court does not recognise as discriminatory precisely the types of attitudes that are so powerful in relation to disabled people – pity and patronisation. This is very similar to the way in which courts have found it difficult to accept as discriminatory attitudes such as paternalism towards women or unconscious racism.

At a deeper level the problem is that disabled people often and obviously, by the very nature of their impairments, possess relevant differences from the rest of the population, and that therefore the formal equality model cannot be applied. American courts have tended to stress that this represents a fundamental distinction between the situation of the disabled and that of other protected groups. Many theorists, while acknowledging the role that discrimination plays in disadvantaging disabled people, stress the uniqueness of their position in similar terms. Burgdorf, one of the architects of the Americans with Disabilities Act, voices a common assumption about the limitations of the parallels which can be drawn with other forms of discrimination: 'The most significant difference between the handicapped and other protected classes is the fact that the condition which initially gives rise to the protected status may also affect performance.'[63]

However, this distinction stems from the formal equality model's conceptualisation of discrimination in terms of individual, intentional acts rather than as structural and systemic. Certainly the continuities with the structural exclusion of women are strong. In that context too we have seen that 'immutable' differences limit the reach of the formal equality model. The chief distinction from the situation of women lies in the scale of structural expenditures which would be required in order to accommodate disabled people to the same extent that able-bodied people are accommodated. This focuses the disputes more squarely on the question of costs.

The fact that disabled people may not be able to perform some jobs does not justify conceptualising their experience of discrimination differently from that of women, since under the equality legislation there is a legal category of jobs from which people can be legitimately excluded, explicitly on the basis of sex. In America, this is termed the 'bona fide occupational qualification' (BFOQ) defence. In Britain the defence is set out in some detail in Section 7 of the Sex Discrimination Act, which provides that discrimination will not be illegal if 'being a man is a genuine occupational qualification for the job'. The Section specifies that this may apply because of physiology, requirements of privacy or decency, because the job involves duties in countries where cultural mores would restrict the performance of those duties by a woman or the job is one of two to be held by a married couple. This authorisation of gender restrictions can therefore apply in a wide variety of circumstances. Whilst the situation with disabled people may be distinguished by the fact that the issue is complicated because different restrictions will apply to different disabilities, or perhaps by the more obvious role of social conventions in validating the discriminatory treatment, neither of these differences stems from a fundamental conceptual distinction.

The Supreme Court has cited with approval a framework for evaluating disability discrimination set out in an article, 'Accommodating the Handicapped',[64] and Ian Bynoe, in the most extensive discussion of disability discrimination legislation yet published in Britain,[65] adopts the same analytical base. This framework places the barriers faced by disabled people into four categories. The first two categories, social bias and the disparate impact of neutral standards, are both experienced by other disadvantaged groups. The other two categories are, in contrast, depicted as unique to disabled people. Surmountable impairment barriers refer to barriers to performance which can be fully overcome with appropriate modifications to the environment; other barriers related to an individual's impairment may be insuperable, even with appropriate modifications.

This last category actually seems to parallel the BFOQ defence in sex discrimination cases, although probably the courts intend it, and would employ it, as a much broader exception. Just as some feminists have criticised the BFOQ defence and pointed out that there is no such exception for racial classifications, I would dispute the validity of creating a legal category of 'insurmountable barriers'. It is based on the social myth of the existence of a hard and fast distinction between ablebodied and disabled people, rather than recognising that people possess a 'spectrum of abilities'.

The leading case referring to 'insurmountable barriers' involved a deaf woman who had been refused entry into a training programme for nurses.[66] The Supreme Court ruled that being deaf presented an insurmountable barrier to becoming a nurse, despite the fact that a number of deaf nurses currently successfully practise in America. This illustrates the danger of including within the framework of discrimination the concept of insurmountable barriers: it is just too tempting for the courts, given the deep-rooted stereotypes about handicapped people, for them to conclude that a case falls within this category.

Just because everyone would not qualify for the Olympics, this does not justify creating a specific legal category, any more than does the fact that not everybody has, for instance, the necessary eyesight to drive. This is not to argue that social restructuring can enable people with disabilities to perform any job. However, especially with the advent of advanced computerised technology, restructuring can enable disabled people to perform most tasks. Where there are jobs which at present no amount of accommodation will allow people with certain disabilities to perform, these people would simply not be regarded as qualified for the job.

Conversely, the concept of surmountable barriers may be useful in considering discrimination against women, as much as for disabled people. The difference with disability discrimination is one of the degree and visibility of the issue rather than rigid distinction. These barriers are structural, and the issue should be presented in terms of how much employers should be made to pay in order to eliminate them.

Disparate impact and disability

McCluskey argues persuasively that the radical interpretation of disparate impact doctrine should be applied to disability discrimination. Identical treatment of disabled and non-disabled people will simply perpetuate the effects of past discrimination if it is not accompanied by modifications to an environment which has been constructed so as to exclude disabled people.

Examining her critique in more detail makes clear the practical advantages of this approach, and in particular the way in which it can be used to reframe the issue of costs. McCluskey's article focuses on the most fiercely contested area of the Rehabilitation Act's anti-discrimination mandate – public transport. The Department of Transportation issued its final regulations implementing s. 504 of the Act in 1986. McCluskey's analysis exposes the able-bodied bias of these rules, which exemplify the assumption that public transport should serve non-disabled people – with the needs of people with disabilities then being treated as an optional extra. In contrast McCluskey, by analysing the situation in terms of a history of prejudice rather than of natural difference, points out that for years disabled people's taxes were used to fund transport that was inaccessible to them, and that therefore some form of compensation is due to them.

The regulations describe inaccessible buses as serving the 'general public', while accessible ones are labelled 'special service vehicles'. The regulations allow local transit services to choose between providing a separate 'special service' system for disabled people or a mixed system. The provision of 'special services' has been widely criticised by disabled people on the basis that it is a form of segregation and inevitably results in inferior services. The regulations specify certain minimum standards for the separate services but add that these standards need not be met if their cost exceeds 3 per cent of the agency's operating budget.

McCluskey points out that these regulations are fundamentally biased, since the cost limit does not apply to the costs of catering to able-bodied people's needs, even when these needs are more burdensome than those of disabled people – for example, seats in buses often cost more than wheelchair securement devices. Moreover, she argues, the cost cap perpetuates past prejudice, since those transit agencies that have made the least effort towards accessible transit in the past are likely to incur the greatest expense in improving access and thus are most likely to be able to employ the cost cap to limit their accessibility expenditure.

Despite the fact that making buses more accessible to disabled people may also benefit a wide range of able-bodied people – small children, elderly people, parents with pushchairs – the rules treat these costs as solely attributable to disabled people. This example vividly illustrates the distortion that is caused by treating disabled people's needs as additional and separate, to be met as a form of charity rather than as part of the common spectrum of human needs.

The disparate impact model in contrast presumes that where a programme has an adverse effect on people with disabilities it is discriminatory and requires remedy, unless this would conflict with 'business necessity'. Although, as we have seen, this term continues to provide a limitation on the scope of change which is required by the anti-discrimination mandate, the transport example illustrates how reframing the question within the disparate impact model can expose biases in the estimation of costs. Thus, McCluskey does not suggest that cost considerations should be totally disregarded, but she does propose several ways of minimising bias. First, courts should closely scrutinise the actual costs of access, as these are often overestimated, and alternatives should be explored to find the least costly. Second, account should be taken of the fact that high costs of access are often the result of past discrimination. Since disabled people have suffered discriminatory treatment in the past, policies which require able-bodied people to incur additional expenses in the future may be justified. Finally, she suggests that cost considerations should be treated at least in an equal fashion for able-bodied and disabled, so that, for instance, any cuts in services should apply to both groups equally.

This analysis succeeds in powerfully reframing the issue of costs with respect to the public provision of services and employment. However, this question becomes more complicated when costs are being imposed on private employers. McCluskey's first two factors remain relevant but the problem remains that courts are reluctant to impose costs on 'innocent' employers. I think Rebell articulates well the concerns which would lead the courts to restrict the application of disparate impact analysis to people with disabilities. He writes in the context of disability that:

A showing of disparate impact cannot automatically justify remedial action because it cannot be presumed to reflect any underlying past or present discriminatory intent ... without some intentionally discriminatory acts to provide a basis for ultimate liability, some further justification is required to establish why an 'innocent' defendant should be put to the trouble or expense of changing practices which 'happen' to cause difficulties for the handicapped ... in the absence of any clear theory of liability or determinable parameter for relief disparate impact analysis as applied to the handicapped is conceptually incomplete.[67]

Indeed, this was precisely the concern expressed by the Supreme Court when considering whether the disparate impact doctrine applied to disability discrimination. As we will see in Chapter 3, the Supreme Court (in *Alexander* v. *Choate*) only reluctantly endorsed this approach for anti-discrimination legislation for people with disabilities. Its reluctance stemmed from the fact that it considered that taking into account the impact of all policies on people with disabilities would be too burdensome, and the Court stressed the need for (without actually providing) firm parameters to the doctrine's scope.

Limits

In practical terms, both the reasonable accommodation and the disparate impact approaches are likely to have limitations imposed on their capacity to remedy structural discrimination because of courts' reluctance to impose the costs of 'social engineering' on 'innocent' employers. The proponents of disparate impact argue that it should be able to achieve more extensive inroads into structural inequalities because its analysis of structural discrimination provides a justification for imposing costs on employers – they are not 'innocent' because they have (albeit unwittingly) participated in the structural exclusion of women/disabled people.

On the other hand, as we have seen, the history of the disparate impact doctrine since Griggs does not really bear out these assertions, since the courts have increasingly exhibited a resistance to imposing any alterations on employers where these would entail significant expense.

The reasonable accommodation approach may in practice possess a greater potential than the disparate impact model for allowing the legislature to lay down clear parameters for anti-discrimination requirements, to which the courts will then be forced to adhere. This framework can also provide alternative criteria for distributing the costs of anti-discrimination, for example ability to pay and number of potential beneficiaries.

Perhaps the relative potential of these two doctrines for achieving substantive change may depend on the relative commitment of courts and legislature to the goal of anti-discrimination. If courts are more disposed to an expansive interpretation of anti-discrimination requirements than the legislature, the more open-ended disparate impact approach will be preferable. However if the judiciary seems to be lagging behind the legislature in its adherence to this goal then the reasonable accommodation approach, because of its potential for providing clear parameters for judicial discretion, may hold greater practical potential, despite its weaker theoretical approach and more stigmatising ideological message.

In part, the way to expand the scope of both doctrinal models is to establish through political struggle the social prioritisation of ending discrimination, and a consequent willingness to accept the costs that this entails. Certainly a firm legislative mandate for extensive and expensive anti-discrimination measures will be helpful in securing a broader impact for them, as will clear and narrow wording of any limitations on employers' liability – whether the limitation takes the form of a requirement that an accommodation be 'reasonable' or of a 'business necessity' defence.

Part of this recognition of the social importance of ending disability discrimination needs to take the form of state subsidies to employers to cover the costs of adapting the work environment. If an employer is to be required to remedy broader historical and social discrimination, the argument goes, s/he should receive some social compensation for this. Courts would be more prepared to order extensive structural alterations if the individual employer were to be reimbursed in some form for the expense incurred.

The Americans with Disabilities Act does this to a certain extent, by making the cost of structural alterations a tax deductible expense. In Britain a system of state subsidies for such adaptations already exists, with payments to interpreters for deaf people and readers for blind people, as well as for physical adaptations and the purchase of additional equipment. This framework of provision would provide an invaluable backing for anti-discrimination legislation.

Such subsidies are important not only in terms of influencing courts' decisions about the extent of alterations which should be imposed by the legislation. They will have a significant impact on the way employers react to these 'burdens'. The Equal Opportunities Commission has complained about the lack of government subsidies for maternity leave, arguing that this will lead to increased discrimination by employers.[68] The same argument will certainly apply to modifications to the work environment for disabled people.

On a more general note, it is important to counter judicial reluctance to impose costs through anti-discrimination legislation, by pointing out other instances where social policies operate in a similar fashion on businesses. An employer's goal of maximising profit is not accepted as a reason for paying less than minimum wages, nor for paying women less than men for equal work. Similarly anti-trust, labour relations and safety laws provide other examples of legislation which imposes costs on employers in the public interest.[69]

Structural alterations

Up to now when discussing the use of law as an agent of social change I have focused exclusively on anti-discrimination laws. An alternative, far more common, legislative approach takes the form of regulations. Directly regulatory legislation imposing structural alterations on all businesses, regardless of the current presence or absence of disabled people, would remove the issue from the individualised, employer/employee tort framework. It has the valuable ideological effect of presenting the issue of cost in social terms and clearly conveys the message that these alterations are required in order to make a discriminatory society accessible to all.

Some broad structural improvements can more readily be achieved for disabled people through blanket requirements of this kind. Where removing barriers is a long-term change, entailing significant expense (such as rendering buildings accessible), these types of structural alterations are the least likely to be achieved by anti-discrimination legislation (whether of the disparate impact or the reasonable accommodation variety), since courts will be reluctant to impose such high costs on 'innocent employers'. Unless the number of affected employees is great, and the employer has substantial resources, individual balancing of their competing interests, such as will inevitably occur within the anti-discrimination framework, is bound to result in the employer's favour.

Not all accommodations are amenable to this approach. Some adjustments are required which specifically fit the individual to the job, for instance by providing aids to enable a particular person to perform a specific job. These individualising accommodations cannot, by definition, be provided prior to an individual applying for a job. However, where access accommodations make the job available to all, and perhaps benefit non-disabled people as well (for instance the installation of ramps or lifts), there may also be cost advantages from the business point of view to achieving structural alterations in this manner. For instance, it is considerably cheaper to implement accessibility while a building is being constructed or other structural alterations are being carried out. In addition, where changes are mandated at the manufacturing stage, economies of scale can be achieved. For example, the National Council on Disability, in its report *Towards Independence*[70] recommended that the federal government use its leverage as a consumer of goods and services to encourage the production of accessible goods and services for people with disabilities. This is potentially a very powerful tool for effecting structural change. Another example of such an approach is the Hearing Aid Compatibility Act 1988, which requires that all new telephones be manufactured so as to be compatible with hearing aids. The Americans with Disabilities Act has addressed a number of alterations to the framework of society in precisely this manner.

From the disabled point of view, legislative mandates for structural alterations may provide a more effective means of achieving extensive changes. Lustgarten and Edwards suggest that such regulatory legislation is more effective, because of severe problems in mobilisation of the legal process, which arise with rights based on forms of law.[71] They argue that anti-discrimination legislation is limited in its effect because it operates by restricting the capacity of the stronger party to a transaction in order to protect the weaker party. The weaker party to a transaction is given rights which can be asserted through litigation. For this law to have an impact, either 'the protected person must invoke the legal process or the penalties must be so credible that the very existence of the law is a goad or a deterrent itself – the in terrorem effect.'[72]

However, the regulatory approach also has its limitations, since the commitment of politicians and bureaucrats to the goal of an accessible and non-discriminatory environment cannot be relied upon to the same extent as the motivations of those directly concerned. The British Building Regulations regarding access for disabled people rely upon the local authorities for their enforcement, and in consequence have a very patchy effect. A situation such as exists in America where, in addition to enforcement by statutory authorities, individuals have the power to sue where they are affected by lack of access, would ensure a greater degree of compliance.

To supplement the systematic reach of regulatory provision with the politically mobilising effect of rights-based legislation would appear to be the most promising combination, and in Chapter 3 we shall see that this is the format of the Americans with Disabilities Act.

Factors external to the workplace – the need for positive rights

Although the assertion of rights is necessary, it is not a sufficient strategy. For all 'minority' groups it is vital that equal rights legislation is supplemented by broader social welfare provision. Finley, in the context of discussing sex equality, criticises the formal equality model for its limited conception of human rights and nature. This model (and, she argues, Western legal jurisprudence generally) conceptualises people as isolated, self-sufficient entities, not recognising their mutual dependence and responsibility for others. She writes that because this understanding of equality searches for the 'irreducible and universal aspects of humanity' it 'requires a focus on sameness and a desire to obliterate differences' and that this involves abstracting individuals from their social context.[73]

Fundamentally this analysis conceives of freedom as the absence of external restraints. It ignores humanity's inevitable interdependence and means that affirmative rights, such as maternity leave, which acknowledge this interdependence are an anomaly.

This argument has particular power in the field of disability. Victor Finklestein attacks the depiction of disabled people as inferior because of their 'dependence' on other people by discussing the fundamental dependence of all people on each other and on socially constructed 'aids'. He gives the example of taps and the whole water supply system as an essential aid to hand washing:

> The fact that an able bodied person requires a washbasin, tap plumbing and so on as well as an army of people to plan build and maintain the water works so that he or she can wash indicates that dependency is not unique to disabled people.[74]

Nor would the use of aids be seen in this context as evidence of inability to carry out a task.

Hahn suggests that 'the European model' is more responsive to affirmative rights. He stresses that Americans, because of their commitment to individualism, understand equality in the particular sense of equality of opportunity.[75] He contrasts the European situation where governments have played a more positive role in determining the allocation of benefits to various portions of the population and alleviating social problems. Certainly most Western European countries embraced the welfare state earlier and with far more commitment than the United States did.

Richard Scotch too states that, compared to Britain, the United States offers relatively less in benefits, and relatively more in protections from discriminatory isolation.

> The American welfare state, initiated in the 1930s and expanded in the 1960s and 1970s has provided far more circumscribed benefits which are also more modest in relation to the overall societal standard of living. British political and legal institutions place much less emphasis on formally defined rights than is the case in the United States.[76]

Hahn regards the European stress on societal responsibility as an important complement to the American emphasis on individual effort in pursuit of the goal of equality. Specifically, he approves European quota systems for people with disabilities and also the widespread provision of government support to compensate disabled people for the additional costs of disability – such as medical care or mobility allowance.

All these analyses stress the importance of an ideological acceptance of social responsibility. Such an acceptance is a necessary basis for any legal approach which accepts that ending discrimination will entail significant disruption and expense. They also suggest the importance of changes in society outside the employment context, for instance childcare/allowance in the case of women, and the provision of facilities for independent living, for example for disabled people. Fundamentally such changes would entail a shift to a means of distributing benefits which is based on neither of the distributive models described by Deborah Stone; that is, based neither on waged labour nor on need defined as dependency. Chapter 7 discusses in more depth the extent to which the requirement for improved welfare policies can be reconciled with, rather than undercut by, disability rights legislation.

3
The Structure of American Laws

This chapter and the next examine the record of American disability rights legislation. Chapter 4 looks at the practical implementation of the law, whilst this chapter focuses on the appropriateness of the legislative structure for addressing the particular issues presented by disability, concentrating on the employment area.

The Americans with Disabilities Act 1990 (ADA) only came into effect in July 1992. However, since its employment provisions are closely modelled on the Rehabilitation Act 1973, it is possible to assess the appropriateness of its provisions through an examination of the courts' interpretations of this earlier Act. It will also be possible to consider the extent to which the ADA improves upon previous legislation and highlight those areas which may form the basis for expanding the scope of this Act's interpretation.

Both Acts are characterised by a structure which balances the goal of non-discrimination against the desire to restrict social cost. The legislation moves substantially beyond the formal equality model, employing the disparate impact, reasonable accommodation and affirmative action approaches, as well as directly mandating enormous structural alterations in society. The dominant approach of both pieces of legislation to the elimination of structural discrimination against disabled people is to require accommodation to the individual's 'special' needs – provided it is not too expensive.

Where the legislation requires widespread, expensive structural alterations the cost of these is spread by phasing them in over time. In addition, by leaving untouched old structures while mandating that future ones be made equally accessible, the overall expense of countering disability discrimination is reduced. Designing an accessible building need not entail significant additional expense, while retrofitting an existing one is considerably more expensive.

Whilst this is clearly a limited approach, I will argue that it does provide a framework in which, through political struggle and creative litigation, the balance can be tilted towards providing greater opportunities for disabled people and reaping greater social benefits.

Rehabilitation Act 1973

Section 504 of the Rehabilitation Act 1973 states that 'no otherwise qualified individual ... shall solely by reason of his handicap be excluded from participation in, be denied benefit of or be subjected to discrimination under any program or activity receiving financial assistance'[1] from the federal government. This section is directly modelled on Title VI of the Civil Rights Act 1964, except for two additional words ('otherwise' and 'solely'), upon which courts would seize at a later date.

Section 503 requires businesses with federal contracts of $2,500 or more to refrain from discrimination and take affirmative action to employ and advance qualified handicapped individuals. Section 501 prohibits handicap discrimination in federal employment and also requires affirmative action.

These provisions have an enormous scope, since they apply to all federally funded employment, education, housing, transport, and health or human services. The significant gains for people with disabilities in the area of higher education, despite fierce opposition from programme recipients, was particularly important.

One powerful effect of the legislation was a requirement that all recipients operate their programmes so that they are readily accessible to, and usable by, disabled persons. Recipients were given three years from the effective date of the regulations to make their programmes accessible. Where facilities were not easily adaptable, programmes could be made accessible by the flexible allocation of activities in accessible parts of buildings. New facilities and, to the maximum extent possible, alterations to existing facilities were to be designed to be readily accessible. These requirements, therefore, represent a typical balancing of the needs of disabled people and attempts to restrict the costs of accommodating them.

Definition of disability

The 1973 Act originally defined 'handicapped' individuals in terms of their impaired capacity to work. Not only did this definition exclude children and elderly people but it also had a self-defeating and stig-matising circularity. At the suggestion of the Office of Civil Rights, the Act was amended in 1974 so that the term 'handicapped' was defined as including anyone:

1) with a physical or mental impairment which substantially limited one or more life activity,
2) with a record of such impairment or
3) regarded as having such an impairment.

This definition establishes prejudice as the defining fact of disability and thus marks the break from the medical to the social model for disability, by locating the 'handicap' in social perceptions and in the restrictions imposed by concrete living situations, rather than listing medical conditions which come into the category of 'disabled'.

As the CQ Researcher noted:

> Although a definition of disability that would yield a precise count (either you're in or you're out) would appease the desire for precision and quantification, experts say it would negate an important component of this public policy: the understanding that disability itself is not always precise and perfectly quantifiable ... A particular disability may limit functioning in one situation, such as riding a bus, while having no impact in another, such as using a word processor.[2]

Definition of discrimination

Discrimination is broadly defined as including practices which directly or indirectly deny opportunities, provide opportunities which are unequal or impose separation.

By defining discrimination as including practices which indirectly deny opportunities to disabled people the regulations suggested that the disparate impact approach would be applied in cases of disability discrimination, just as it is in race and sex discrimination cases. However, outside the issue of selection criteria in which the regulations explicitly set out the implications of this approach, this proved to be a particularly controversial area of interpretation, with conflicting opinions in the lower courts only being resolved by the Supreme Court in 1984. The case of *Alexander* v. *Choate*[3] (discussed in more detail below) ruled that the disparate impact analysis did apply to the Rehabilitation Act, but suggested that its application would be restricted. This approach was not utilised in employment litigation, nor was it discussed during the legislative history of the ADA, so its broader potential remains unexplored.

The regulations do, however, employ the disparate impact model with regard to selection criteria for employment (the area in which it has been chiefly utilised in race and sex discrimination cases). Recipients are prohibited from using criteria or methods of administration which have the effect of discrimination, whether or not they have the intent to discriminate. Selection criteria which screen out disabled individuals must be job related and consistent with business necessity.

The regulations interpret the Act as requiring more than formal equality; they use the 'special treatment' approach, discussed in Chapter 2. The ability of an individual with a disability to participate must be assessed in the context of the 'essential' goals of an employment position (or programme or service), which need not necessarily coincide with the manner that such positions have been structured or performed in the past. Consideration must be given to alternative methods of achieving the essential tasks of the job or programme, which would allow the participation of the disabled applicant. Thus handicapped applicants are regarded as qualified (and therefore entitled under the statute to protection from discrimination) if they can perform the essential functions of the job or programme with reasonable accommodation, unless such accommodation would cause undue hardship.

An interesting departure from the formal equality/equal treatment model is the fact that the Rehabilitation Act does not forbid discrimination against non-disabled persons. The Civil Rights Act 1964 bans discrimination on the basis of race and sex, and therefore extends as much protection to the dominant groups as to groups who are oppressed by those groups. Nor is this merely a theoretical nicety. White men have made extensive use of the Civil Rights Act both to block affirmative action programmes and to break into previously female dominated areas. This colour/gender blind approach perpetuates the notion that racism and sexism are constituted by random individual acts rather than an understanding that such acts draw force from structural power differences in society. When the ADA was being debated there was no serious proposal that such an approach should be applied to disability, probably because of the acceptance that extensive positive action or 'special' measures of differential treatment would be required to give any reality to equal opportunities to disabled people.

Americans with Disabilities Act 1990

Title I: Employment

All employers with over 15 employees are prohibited from discriminating against a 'qualified individual with a disability'. (These employment provisions only applied to employers with 25 or more employees prior to July 1994.) The employment section of the ADA is explicitly and closely modelled on the Rehabilitation Act, so that the definitions generally follow those contained in the regulations implementing the earlier Act. Thus the definition of disability remains identical to that used in the implementation of the Rehabilitation Act, as does the definition of discrimination, which requires reasonable accommodation to the known physical or mental limitations of an otherwise qualified individual with a disability (unless to do so would cause undue hardship), and the use of non-discriminatory selection criteria.

However, the legislature did correct some of the ambiguities which had impaired the effectiveness of the earlier measure. Thus there is no requirement here, as in the Rehabilitation Act, that discrimination must be 'solely' on the basis of disability. In addition a 'qualified individual' with a disability is explicitly defined as one who with or without reasonable accommodation can perform the essential functions of the job. This resolved considerable judicial disputes concerning this point under the Rehabilitation Act.

The limited application of the Act to employers of 15 or more employees is a concession to 'small' businesses and not logically required to limit the costs imposed on them, since the undue hardship defence could be invoked to limit any expense. It seems wrong in principle for small businesses to remain free blatantly to discriminate against employees (but not against customers where they provide 'public accommodations'). In Britain, where small businesses comprise a significant proportion of the economy, such an exemption would need to be opposed.

Non-employment provisions

The scope of the provisions in the ADA regarding issues other than employment is enormous. They mandate huge structural alterations in society, albeit phased in over the next 30 years. In a sense the transport provisions are more radical than the employment provisions, since these are uniformly required, rather than triggered by the presence of a disabled individual. Their impact in facilitating the integration of disabled people into mainstream society cannot be overemphasised. Newly constructed public facilities will be equally radically altered.

Titles II and III: Public accommodations and services

Titles II and III of the Act ban discrimination in public services and accommodations. Public accommodations were not covered by the Rehabilitation Act, except in so far as they were federally funded. Discrimination in these contexts is defined in accordance with the basic approach of the Rehabilitation Act. New public accommodations and commercial facilities must be readily accessible, unless it is structurally impractical to do so. All alterations must be accessible. The architectural standards for accessibility in new construction and alterations are contained in guidelines issued by the Architectural and Transportation Compliance Board, an independent federal agency.

Existing structures must be altered to render them accessible, where such modifications are 'readily achievable', which is defined as easily accomplished without much expense (factors such as the size of the company and type of business will be taken into account). If the removal of the architectural barriers is not readily achievable, the goods or services must be provided through alternative methods where doing so is readily achievable.

Operators of public accommodations may not impose eligibility criteria that operate to screen out individuals with disabilities unless they are necessary in order to provide goods and services. It is also dis-criminatory to fail to make 'readily achievable' modifications in practice, where these would enable people with disabilities to have access to and use of public accommodations; nor can goods or services be denied because of the absence of auxiliary aids, unless providing such aids would fundamentally alter the nature of the good or service or result in an undue burden.

Title IV: Transport

Public transport was widely affected by the Rehabilitation Act, and was the most fiercely contested arena, with extensive court battles and street demonstrations. Section 504 of the Rehabilitation Act, requiring recipients of federal funds to operate in a non-discriminatory way, applied to most public transport companies. As with other areas of provision, regulations were promulgated stipulating in detail what 'non-discrimination' entailed. However, successive regulations were challenged in the courts, by both disability activists and the transport companies (see Chapter 4).

Since the interpretation of the simple non-discriminatory mandate had been shown to be too open to conflicting interpretations, the ADA's approach was to set out in detail the requirements for non-discrimi-natory transport, together with a timetable for their implementation. Title IV of the ADA requires all new buses to be accessible, and public transport companies that buy new buses, rail or other vehicles must ensure that they are accessible to people with disabilities. New public transport facilities must also be readily accessible. Although there is no general requirement that existing facilities be made accessible, if any alterations are carried out these must be executed in such a way that the altered sections are accessible.

Commuter rail stations must be made accessible within three years. Commuter services must have at least one passenger car per train which is accessible within five years of enactment. Inter-city rail carriers must be made accessible as soon as practicable, with a time limit of 29 years.

Private transport businesses must, in future, only purchase or lease accessible vehicles. For 'small providers' the time limit for implemen-tation of this provision is seven years, while for larger businesses it is six years. Where transport agencies supplement inaccessible mainstream services with 'special' paratransit systems (the equivalent of the British 'Dial-A-Ride' systems), these must provide a comparable service to that provided to the general public.

The detailed provisions for both private and public transport were a tremendous achievement for the disabled activists who had struggled to achieve accessible public transport under the Rehabilitation Act. The only victory for the powerful transport lobby was to have the provisions phased in over a period of 30 years. But the principal of equal and integrated transport for disabled people is clearly stated in the Act.

Title V: Telecommunication
By 1993 telephone companies were required to provide telecommunication relay systems throughout their service areas on a full-time basis. This is another provision of enormous symbolic and practical importance, achieved after deaf activists had achieved international prominence through their struggles. It establishes a fundamental structural alteration in the operation of society. These provisions are required as a matter of course, and therefore many more jobs will become accessible without the necessity of 'reasonable accommodation'.

Before considering the effectiveness of the Rehabilitation Act, given the constraints in which it operated, I will examine in some detail the operation of its legal categories, to determine the extent to which they succeeded in capturing the mechanisms of disability discrimination. I will focus on the area of employment.

The legislation in action

The Supreme Court decisions concerning the substantive meaning of the Rehabilitation Act not only highlights some crucial interpretative issues, but also provides an insight into the development of judicial appreciation of the nature of disability discrimination. I shall therefore briefly examine the three leading Supreme Court opinions in this area before proceeding to a more systematic analysis of how effective the legislation has been in practice.

Supreme Court decisions
The first case under Section 504 to reach the Supreme Court, *Southeastern Community College* v. *Davis*,[4] highlighted one of the key issues in the interpretation of the Rehabilitation Act, how the phrase 'otherwise qualified' should be interpreted. If it meant that applicants must be qualified for the job in every respect except for their possession of a disability which has no effect on their ability to perform the job, then there would be no requirement for employers to provide reasonable accommodation. On the other hand, if 'otherwise qualified' meant qualified apart from the disability, then the non-discrimination mandate of the Rehabilitation Act might also include a reasonable accommodation requirement. All the federal regulations defined 'qualified' as including consideration of whether reasonable accommodation would enable the applicant to perform the job or participate in the programme. However, many of the lower courts had overruled the regulations on this point.

Davis was a hearing impaired practical nurse who sought admission to Southeastern's nursing degree programme. She was rejected because of her hearing impairment. The college argued that she could not safely practise her chosen profession nor satisfactorily participate in the clinical section of the programme without extensive modification of the programme. The Court found that the college's refusal did not constitute unlawful discrimination, since it could not be obliged to modify the programme to such an extent that it constituted a 'fundamental alteration in the nature of the program'.[5] The Court pointed out that while s. 501 and s. 503 explicitly required affirmative action, s. 504 did not. It thus came close to interpreting the anti-discrimination mandate in s. 504 as merely requiring 'equal treatment' and equating any alterations to programmes with affirmative action.

At one point the opinion states ominously:

If these regulations were to require substantial adjustments in existing programs beyond those necessary to eliminate discrimination against otherwise qualified individuals they would do more than clarify the meaning of s. 504. Instead they would constitute an unauthorized extension of the obligations imposed by that statute ... We do not argue that the line between a lawful refusal to extend affirmative action and illegal discrimination against handicapped persons always will be clear. It is possible to envision situations where an insistence on continuing past requirements or practices might arbitrarily deprive genuinely qualified handicapped persons of the opportunity to participate in a covered program. Technological advances can be expected to enhance opportunities to rehabilitate the handicapped or otherwise qualify them for useful employment. Such advances also may enable attainment of these goals without imposing undue financial or administrative burdens upon a state. Thus situations may arise where a refusal to modify an existing program might become unreasonable and discriminatory.[6]

This section of the opinion reflects the medical model of disability, seeing the individual's incapacities rather than the social context as the problem. It seems to be suggesting that the solution to the social exclusion of disabled people is a cure which will stop them being disabled, rather than ending social discrimination.

Although confused and ambivalent about the requirement of reasonable accommodation, the Court did make some attempt to apply the narrow, formal equality approach. It looked beyond the broad exclusionary classification, examining the degree and nature of Davis' deafness. Nevertheless, its constrained understanding of discrimination meant that the opinion is itself both an example of prejudice as applied to the particular facts of the case, and ambiguously uncertain with regard to broader principles. The Court failed to perform a proper job analysis to show that the clinical skills required for programme completion were related to successful performance in the nursing positions for which the programme prepared students. It also failed adequately to address the question of whether the programme could be altered reasonably to accommodate Davis. It noted that regulations did not require the provision of an interpreter and therefore did not undertake any analysis of the reliability or costs of the plaintiff's proposals either to provide individual supervision or waive the clinical requirements – possibly accompanied by a restriction on her practising certificate.

In effect the Court concluded that deaf people could not be nurses. This conclusion is contradicted by the fact that deaf people are successfully employed as nurses. For example a Civil Service Commission survey, completed shortly after this case, revealed 150 hearing impaired nurses employed by the federal government.

After intensive educational efforts by disability rights lawyers (using procedural mechanisms such as amicus curae briefs, described in Chapter 5) the Court later revised its views on what constituted discrimination, and the consequent requirement for reasonable accommodation, and in so doing showed a greater insight into the problems faced by disabled people. The unanimous decision in *Alexander* v. *Choate* represents the extent of this transformation. The contrasts between the two unanimous decisions of the Court are striking: *Davis* minimised the significance of the regulations, while *Alexander* gave great credence to these federal agency interpretations; *Davis* promoted a narrow interpretation of the Act while *Alexander*, by its acceptance of some forms of disparate impact, encouraged a broad interpretation.

The issue presented in *Alexander* v. *Choate* was whether disparate impact discrimination was prohibited by s. 504, regardless of the existence of intentional discrimination. The plaintiff challenged the decision of Tennessee Medicaid to reduce cover for in-hospital days from 20 to 14 per year, on the basis that it had a discriminatory impact on disabled patients who, as a class, required more in-patient days than non-disabled patients. The Court upheld the decision on the basis that this particular disparate impact was not discriminatory because state medicaid did not have to provide adequate health care, merely meaningful access to health care. Consequently the handicapped were given equal access to the benefit of the programme, since they were provided with meaningful access to health care.

Although the Court did not accept that this particular instance of disparate impact was discriminatory, it did hold that this doctrine would be applicable to disability discrimination in some instances. 'Discrimination against the handicapped was perceived by Congress to be most often the product not of invidious animus but rather of thoughtlessness and indifference – of benign neglect',[7] and therefore a requirement to prove intent would mean that anti-discrimination law would not be able to reach many instances of discrimination. The opinion points out, for instance, that architectural barriers would not be removed if it was necessary to show discriminatory intent.

The Court was reluctant, however, to conclude that all disparate impacts were discriminatory per se:

> Because the handicapped are typically not similarly situated to the non-handicapped, such a stance would in essence require each recipient of federal funds first to evaluate the effects on handicapped persons of every proposed action that might touch the interest of the handicapped and then consider alternatives for achieving the same objectives with less severe disadvantages for the handicapped. The formalizing of this process could lead to a wholly unwieldy administration and adjustive burden.[8]

The opinion argued that two countervailing considerations are involved: a requirement to end discrimination and the 'desire to keep s. 504 within manageable bounds'.[9] (This seems to beg the question, 'whose desire?') However the Court, not very helpfully, limited its considerations to the particular case and avoided drawing any broader guidelines for the parameters of disparate impact in disability cases.

There have been few cases which have sought to explore the implications of disparate impact in the employment context, both because of the reluctance and uncertainty exhibited by the courts in this area, and because the reasonable accommodation mandate effectively dominates the legal response to the issues.

This opinion contains another significant advance upon the previous one. It delicately corrects the *Davis* decision's confusion regarding reasonable accommodation and whether it constituted a form of affirmative action.

> Our use of the term affirmative action in this context has been severely criticized for failing to appreciate the difference between affirmative action and reasonable accommodation; the former is said to refer to a remedial policy for the victims of past discrimination while the latter relates to the elimination of existing obstacles against the handicapped. Regardless of the aptness of our choice of words in Davis it is clear from the context ... that the term affirmative action referred to those changes, adjustments and modifications to existing programs that would be substantial ... rather than to those changes which would be reasonable accommodations.[10]

The most recent Supreme Court case concerning s. 504, *School Board of Nassau County, Florida* v. *Arline*,[11] involved a schoolteacher discharged after a relapse of tuberculosis. The school board argued that Arline was dismissed not because of diminished physical capacities but because of the threat of contagion, and that this therefore did not constitute discrimination on the basis of disability. The Court did not accept this distinction. It argued that such an approach would mean that those accused of being contagious had no opportunity to have their cases examined in the light of medical evidence to see if they were 'otherwise qualified'. The opinion represents the clearest yet judicial understanding of the force of discrimination faced by disabled people and a powerful statement of s. 504's principles and application to the particular facts: Congress acknowledged that society's accumulated myths and fears about disability and disease are as handicapping as the physical limitations that flow from actual impairment.'[12] The opinion stated that Congress aimed to protect the handicapped 'not only from simple prejudice, but from "archaic attitudes and laws" and from "the fact that the American people are simply unfamiliar with and insensitive to the difficulties confronting individuals with handicaps"'.[13]

The Court assumed without discussion that s. 504 required reasonable accommodation, and stated that an individualised inquiry was necessary for the school board to ascertain whether Arline was 'otherwise qualified', that is whether she was contagious and, if so, whether reasonable accommodation could eliminate the risk. The Court was thus clear that the possibility of reasonable accommodation should be considered in deciding whether or not the person is 'otherwise qualified'. It specified that when rejecting a handicapped person on the grounds of safety the enquiry needed to consider the nature, duration and severity of the risk, and the probability of transmission.

How adequately has disability discrimination been addressed by the legislation?

Discrimination against disabled people involves the same basic modes of operation as sex and race discrimination. I examine these processes below under the following headings: individual bias, exclusionary classifications, neutral practices and structural barriers. Apart from the final category, which courts have sought to address by the concept of reasonable accommodation to an extent which they have not been willing to apply in cases of sex, race or religious discrimination, the courts have generally held that the jurisprudential framework developed under Title VII of the Civil Rights Act 1964 is equally applicable to discrimination against people with disabilities.

Individual bias

This form of discrimination involves treating people who are disabled adversely without any rational reason or pretext. That is to say it represents a form of 'pure' prejudice, where the employer is not arguing that the disabled people cannot perform the necessary tasks, just that s/he does not want them around. In the past this form of discrimination has been both frequent and explicit. It is the type of prejudice which most conforms with the popular understanding of discrimination, and the formal equality model.

In the case of *Smith* v. *Barton* [14] (involving, ironically, applicants for the position of Chief of Rehabilitation Services) the Appeal Court commented, 'this case is unusual in that the defendants disavow any reliance on the plaintiffs' handicap',[15] observing that most cases have alleged that handicap rendered the person unsuitable for the job. Another court concluded that such cases did not raise any issues that were unique to the disabled situation, and that the method of analysis and burdens of proof and production employed in other Title VII cases should apply.[16] A prima facie case can be established by the plaintiff showing that s/he has applied for a position for which s/he was qualified and 'was rejected under circumstances indicating discrimination on the basis of an impermissible factor'.[17]

The burden then shifts to the defendant to rebut the presumption of discrimination by producing evidence that the plaintiff was rejected for a legitimate, non-discriminatory reason. If the defendant does so the burden then shifts back to the plaintiff to show that 'the proffered reason was not the true reason for the decision'.[18]

Amy Gittler comments on the extra problems which 'handicapped' people may face in cases involving individual allegations of discrimination because of the absence of statistics.[19] Statistics showing the discrepancy between the percentage of a protected class in the general population (or, where the job involves specific skills, in that particular labour pool) and the percentage of employees that are in that class are often used in America to show a pattern of discrimination by an employer, and to strengthen the suggestion that the employer's proffered reason for rejecting the applicant is pretextual. Such statistics have also been used in the context of a class action to show patterns of discrimination against members of a protected class.

Such data simply does not exist for the disabled population, and even if it did the issue is complicated because of the variety of disabilities and degrees of impairment within disability categories:

> The fact that an employer employs 15 epileptics is not necessarily probative of whether he or she has discriminated against a blind person ... an employer may attempt to create the appearance of compliance with the law by employing several epileptics, or cured

cancer patients, while at the same time refusing to hire the more visibly and severely handicapped.[20]

Thus, the only relevant statistical sample for these purposes would be one which relates to persons in the recruitment area, with the particular disability of the applicant, who possess any necessary qualifications. Even if disparities could be shown between the employment statistics of the employer and the relevant labour pool, 'such statistical analyses would be so small as to have little legal significance'.[21]

Gittler's other criticism of the use of statistics in this context is very telling:

> The data will always show that few if any handicapped are currently employed by the defendant employer compared to the numbers of handicapped in the overall population ... if the statistics were given the same weight for handicapped persons as they were for blacks or women, the handicapped plaintiff would always prevail.[22]

However, Yellin has more belief in the value of statistical data in this area.[23] He suggests that the Equal Employment Opportunity Commission (EEOC) should see part of its enforcement responsibility as the collection of such statistics, and proposes a survey to estimate the interactions between impairments and working conditions in the contemporary economy. This would be valuable not only for vocational guidance, but also to alert employers to those situations where minor modifications of the physical environment would enable disabled employees to work. Such information could also provide the statistical basis for establishing discrimination – for instance where disabled workers form a disproportionate percentage of redundancies.

As the other possible avenues of defence are reduced and the extent of the employer's obligations under the reasonable accommodation requirement are extended, it seems likely that more employers will seek to avoid their obligation to accommodate and otherwise cease discriminating, by alleging that factors other than handicap were responsible for their decision. Such cases of covert discrimination, so common in the sex and race arena, will become more frequent.

Exclusionary classifications

A blanket exclusion, based on inaccurate generalisations about the abilities of certain categories of disabled people (for example where blind or deaf people are explicitly barred from occupations), is the type of discrimination which next approximates to the formal equality conception of discrimination. Such classifications will be found unacceptable if they stem from inaccurate generalisations or stereotypes:

although a group may, on average, possess or lack certain relevant qualities, this may not be the case with an individual member of the group. The need for 'individualisation' is particularly important because of the 'spectrum of abilities', discussed in Chapter 1. Such classifications may also be discriminatory because they do not actually correspond to the physical or mental requirements of the job.

Exclusionary classification cases involving people with disabilities turn on the same principles as sex discrimination cases where the employer explicitly excludes women or men from a category of employment, regardless of an individual's qualifications or abilities. Title VII provides that such exclusions can only by valid if the employer proves that sex is a bona fide occupational qualification (BFOQ). The particular characteristics which the excluded class lacks must be necessary for the performance of the job, and the aspects of the job for which the BFOQ is claimed must embody the essence or the purpose of the business.

For such categories to be upheld in sex discrimination cases, the Court in *Weeks* v. *Southern Bell Telephone & Telegraph Company*[24] held that the employer must prove that 'all or substantially all [members of the protected class] would be unable to perform safely and efficiently the duties of the job involved'.[25]

Under the Rehabilitation Act courts have questioned, or invalidated as overly broad, exclusionary classifications based on blindness,[26] epilepsy,[27] learning disabilities[28] and multiple sclerosis.[29] On the other hand, some courts have been prepared to uphold such classifications even though they were based on assumptions rather than solid evidence.[30] To a certain extent this is the result of ignorance, which it is hoped increasing familiarity with disability law, and the details of particular disabilities, will remedy.

Courts have been particularly likely to give broad deference to employers' judgements where safety issues are involved or where individualised assessments would entail an administrative burden. There was a suggestion in the Supreme Court case of *Southeastern Community College* v. *Davis* that such an undue administrative burden might justify a blanket exclusion rather than individualised accommodation. However, this proposal has not been taken up in the majority of decisions. For instance, in *Costner* v. *United States*[31] a federal District Court rejected the contention that the US Department of Transportation lacked the resources or personnel to make an individualised determination of whether a person with epilepsy that is under control can safely operate a motor vehicle. 'Such inconvenience should not stand in the way of justice.'[32] This approach reflects decisions in sex and race discrimination cases. The Supreme Court case of *School Board* v. *Arline*[33] seems to consolidate the requirement for the employer to conduct an individualised enquiry rather than make speculative decisions based on misinformed health and safety claims.

Neutral practices

To avoid discrimination on the basis of disability it is important not only to assess accurately the individual's capacities rather than employing stereotypes, but also to scrutinise closely the requirements of the job to see whether these can be met by those capacities. Concepts of ability or disability have no meaning except in the context of a particular task or activity. 'Not all physical or mental differences cause functional impairments, and not all functional impairments restrict activities, and not all activity restrictions cause vocational ... limitations.'[34]

The Rehabilitation Act regulations (and subsequently the ADA) adopt the disparate impact approach originating in Title VII jurisprudence. Although this could theoretically be employed in a broad-reaching, radical strategy (as described in Chapter 2), the only issue which the Rehabilitation Act regulations, or indeed the ADA, explicitly addresses from this perspective is the legitimacy of selection criteria. (This is also the issue to which the approach has largely been confined in sex and race cases.) Such criteria may discriminate against people with disabilities by either inaccurately measuring abilities, or accurately measuring abilities but inaccurately correlating them with activities.

Some employers specify certain physical or mental requirements in effect as a substitute for exclusionary classifications, for example a requirement for 20/20 vision or a certain blood sugar level. The employer in *Bentivegna* v. *US Department of Labor*,[35] the city of Los Angeles, had imposed a selection criterion requiring 'controlled' blood sugar levels. The acknowledged goal of this criterion was to screen out people with diabetes unless their condition was controlled at certain blood sugar levels. This requirement was not linked to any particular job but was defended on the basis that such people had a greater risk of long-term health problems. The Court refused to allow such a defence:

> Potentially troublesome health problems will affect a large proportion of the handicapped population. Consistent attendance and an expectation of continuity will be important to any employer. Such considerations cannot provide the basis for discriminatory job qualifications unless they can be connected directly to 'business necessity' or safe performance of the job.[36]

This ruling will prove extremely important in curbing some of the excesses of health screening described in Chapter 1.

In other cases an unthinking social bias rather than conscious exclusion operates. For instance, some employers may screen out people with certain disabilities by using tests which fail to measure accurately the qualities genuinely required for the job. One successfully contested case involved a written test for a plant operator. The applicant, because of his dyslexia, could not pass the test, but succeeded in having it invalidated in court.[37] The ADA explicitly bans such practices.[38]

Both the Rehabilitation Act and the ADA protect from discrimination those individuals who, 'with or without reasonable accommodation, can perform the essential functions of the employment position that such individuals hold or desire'.[39] Aside from the issue of reasonable accommodation, which I will consider below, the analysis logically breaks down into two parts – what are the essential functions of a job, and are the selection criteria employed legitimate? A related issue, which employers often adduce, is that of safety of the individuals concerned.

Essential functions

This term is not defined in the Rehabilitation Act regulations, and courts have only infrequently dealt with the issue. One commentator has argued, with regard to the Rehabilitation Act, that:

> Because there is no strictly analytical way to decide which functions are essential to a particular job, such a determination depends upon how one defines both the purposes of the job in question and the permissible goals of employers. The inability of an employee to perform any given task will impose costs on an employer ... The only real issue is how great a cost an employer should bear. The regulations cast this political question into a fictive quest for essential and non-essential job functions.[40]

This term is not defined in the ADA, although (as a result of lobbying by business interests) it provides that considerable weight should be given to the employer's analysis of job requirements. The Senate Labor Committee report for the ADA stated that essential functions were those which were fundamental and not marginal, and in practice this requires employers to evaluate job tasks in some detail. This is likely to be a contested area of interpretation.

Legitimacy of selection criteria

The next question is whether the selection criteria are legitimate. Selection criteria which screen out disabled people will be discriminatory unless they can be shown to be related to the essential requirements of the position in question and to be consistent with business necessity. Given the extensive litigation under the Civil Rights Act with regard to business necessity this is also likely to be an area of intense legal struggle. In *Bentivegna* v. *US Department of Labor* the Court set a promising precedent:

> The importance of preserving job opportunities for the handicapped sets a high standard for the effectiveness of job qualifications that adversely affect disabled people ... the courts must be wary that business necessity is not confused with mere expediency. If a job qualification is to be permitted to exclude handicapped individuals, it must be directly connected with, and must substantially promote business necessity and safe performance.[41]

Safety

Safety issues may be raised to disqualify a disabled person from employment. Case law under the Rehabilitation Act established that an employer could not refuse employment to people on the basis that they were putting themselves at risk. The Court in *Pushkin* v. *Regents of the University of Colorado*[42] noted that such paternalism was a common form of discrimination against disabled people, 'under the guise of extending a helping hand or a mistaken, restrictive belief as to the limitations of a handicapped person'. Or, as another court expressed it: 'The purpose of s504 is to permit handicapped individuals to live life as fully as they are able, without paternalistic authorities deciding that certain activities are too risky for them.'[43] It is for individuals themselves to evaluate any risks attached to employment.

Under the ADA employers are provided with a defence to charges of discrimination if they can establish that an individual poses 'a direct threat to the health or safety of other individuals in the workplace'.[44] It is significant that no mention is made of individuals endangering their own health.

When the health and safety of others is the prime consideration the factors listed in the Supreme Court case of *School Board* v. *Arline* should be considered, that is the decision should be based on facts concerning the nature, severity and duration of the risk and (where contagious diseases are involved) the probability that the disease will be transmitted. The Court did not specify the weight that should be attributed to the different factors, and the danger with such a formulation is that where the nature of the harm is greatly feared (such as with AIDS) this might be allowed to outweigh the slightness of the risk of transmission.

Structural barriers

As discussed in previous chapters, structural discrimination arises from the fact that tasks and workplaces have been constructed for able-bodied people, and as a result may be unsuitable for a disabled person without some form of alteration. Often only a simple reorganisation of the workplace or tasks is required, which can be achieved with little expense. However, other alterations may entail considerable cost. The question of how much employers are required to spend to make their employment accessible will undoubtedly be the most fiercely disputed area under the new Act.

Reasonable accommodation

The two central terms employed in both Acts for addressing the removal of structural barriers from employment are 'reasonable accommodation' and 'undue hardship'. Neither term is definitively defined by the statutes, and the regulations interpreting both Acts merely illustrate the meaning of reasonable accommodation by giving a list of examples.

In practice, therefore, the determination of whether or not a specific accommodation is required hinges on the issue of whether or not it entails undue hardship. This is defined in the ADA as 'an action requiring significant difficulty or expense when considered in the light of'[45] a list of factors: the type of business (including the structure of the workforce, and the geographical, administrative and fiscal relationship of a particular facility within a multisite business), number of employees and the budget of the business (and of the specific facility involved), and the nature and cost of the accommodations involved.

This means of limiting the extent of the anti-discrimination requirement proved unsatisfactory under the Rehabilitation Act. One commentator criticised these terms as revolving around 'an ambiguous list of unweighted characteristics'.[46] Certainly under the Rehabilitation Act these factors were given widely varying emphasis, and more than one court expressed its frustration at the confused way in which the issue is posed. The Court in *Prewitt* v. *US Postal Service* [47] noted that the term reasonable accommodation had first arisen on cases involving religious discrimination (such as Sabbatarians seeking accommodation to enable them to refrain from working on certain days). The Civil Rights Act 1964 requires employers to accommodate such practices unless to do so would involve undue hardship. The Supreme Court interpreted this requirement as not extending beyond an accommodation at 'de minimis cost'[48] – that is requiring no more than minimal expenditure. However, in *Prewitt* v. *US Postal Service* the Court concluded that such an interpretation of 'undue hardship' would not be appropriate in the disability context: 'Congress clearly intended the federal government to take measures that would involve more than de minimis cost'.

Nelson v. *Thornborough* [49] contains a more detailed consideration of the parameters of reasonable accommodation. This case involved several blind employees of the Department of Public Works (DPW), where changes in the requirements of the job (from social work to form filling) had led the group of employees to increased reliance on a reader. They were claiming that the employer should meet this cost or acquire aids such as a braille manual or computer equipment which would alleviate the need for a reader. The Court described the concept of 'reasonable accommodation' as a 'quasi-legislative compromise between competing interests', stressing that:

> The proper resolution of the case cannot be deduced from the words of the statute, but must instead represent a quantitative judgment ... Thus arguments over otherwise qualified, reasonable accommodation, undue hardship and affirmative action all collapse into one issue: would the cost of providing part-time readers be greater than the Act allows?[50]

In this case the Court held that, despite budgetary cutbacks, the employer was sufficiently large (noting that the DPW allocated $600,000 for travel reimbursements for employees alone) that it would not be an undue hardship for it to provide the requested accommodation.

In a footnote the Court commentated:

> It is worth noting ... that the DPW considers employable and thus ineligible for benefits, handicapped applicants for public assistance who are 'fully employable with reasonable accommodation' – reasonable accommodation being defined for this purpose as 'structural modifications, modified work schedules, acquisition of modified equipment or devices, provision of readers or interpreters, job restructuring and similar actions.' It does not seem wholly unfair to impose upon DPW the same requirements that DPW imposes upon its clients and their would-be employers.[!][51]

Other cases also imposed substantial modifications. For example, one involving nursing staff with epilepsy required their employer to provide additional supervision or, where necessary, assign staff to clerical positions.[52] However, another strand of cases treated the question less favourably for the disabled plaintiff. For example, one court held that the cost to the Post Office of accommodating an individual with a step stool and assistance would result in a loss of efficiency which would entail undue hardship.[53]

It is difficult to resist the conclusion that the 'courts use undue hardship as a label for any accommodation that they have already decided not to require in a given case. Courts have thus developed idiosyncratic, fact specific rules without precedential value.'[54]

The concept that there should be some financial limitation upon the requirement for modifications is inherent in this piecemeal approach to adapting the work environment for disabled people. Commentators from both sides have criticised the vagueness of these standards. The *Wall Street Journal* was merely one of a number of voices describing the ADA as 'an employment Act for lawyers'.[55] The ambiguities of these core definitions are at least partly responsible for the widely diverging estimates of the financial effects of the legislation, with supporters of the measure arguing that the costs of compliance would be 'no big deal',[56] and opponents claiming that it would 'send businesses down the chute'.[57]

In practice, the woolliness of the definitions is probably most dangerous for plaintiffs, given the continued dominance of the formal equality model and consequent judicial reluctance to impose costs on employers by requiring significant alterations. This risk is compounded by the continuing prevalence of stereotypes and bias against disabled people, amongst jurists as much as the population at large. The danger is that in the absence of substantive categories judges will fill the gap with their own intuitive assessments. 'This process is likely to be influenced by prevalent normative assumptions about the meaning of work and by familiar images of particular jobs and arrangements of workplaces.'[58]

The original draft of the ADA attempted to employ a much stricter reasonable accommodation/undue hardship test: employers would have to provide accommodation unless this would have threatened the existence of a business. The watering down of this standard was a crucial area of compromise for achieving the successful passage of the Act.

A number of other suggestions have been proffered by commentators to facilitate the achievement of consistent standards. Steven Gerse[59] has suggested that financial restrictions on the costs of accommodations be eliminated, and employers required to provide whatever accommodations are needed by disabled employees. However, he justifies this in the context of the Rehabilitation Act on the basis that contractors and programme operators are recipients of federal funds, and it is therefore very unlikely that such a standard would ever be imposed on the private sector employers covered by the ADA. His alternative proposal, if some limit is required, is for an upper limit to expenditure based on a percentage of the operating budget or the wages bill.

In Chapter 2 I concluded that disabled applicants would be best served by an explicit reconciliation, such as Gerse proposes, of the goals of full, non-discriminatory participation by disabled people in society and the limitation of the economic costs of restructuring in order to protect profits. A more quantitative standard would place valuable constraints on judicial discretion.

The proposal that the maximum cost limit for an accommodation be related to the level of an employee's salary was explicitly rejected during the debates on the ADA, because of the historically low wage levels of disabled workers. Suggestions that a limit on the cost of accommodation should be related to an employer's ability to pay, assessed by a combination of profitability (this by itself is too prone to fluctuation from one year to another), budget and assets, seems the most promising approach. The long-term advantages of any modifications to other employees and customers, both able-bodied and disabled, should also be taken into account, as should an understanding that all employees require a level of accommodation. The example of a wheelchair user who might require a desk to be lowered but would not require a chair to be purchased most immediately comes to mind. The extent to which an employer is entitled to have the costs of accommodation reimbursed by the federal government should also be part of the equation. The courts are likely to be much more willing to impose expensive requirements on employers if all or part of these will not be met by the individual employer, but by the government as a social cost.

In summary, certain key issues remain to be determined through litigation and, if necessary, through future amendments to the Act. The interpretation of the concepts 'reasonable accommodation', 'undue hardship', 'essential functions' and 'business necessity' will determine to a great extent the ultimate reach of the legislation. An expansive interpretation, promoting the ending of disability discrimination, can be supported by reference to the clear analysis of discrimination contained in the legislative history of the ADA. However, those seeking to restrict the scope of the Act might quote the argument put forward by some proponents of the Act that changes would not entail significant expense. It is crucial that the issue of costs is firmly placed within the broader perspective discussed by Martha McCluskey.[60]

One final comment on the implementation of the legislation within the courts. Opponents of the ADA played heavily on the supposed looseness of its definitions, which, it was alleged, would provide a goldmine for lawyers. On the evidence of the Rehabilitation Act this will be far from the case. The definition of disability proved very easy to put into practice, with only a very few cases exploring borderline issues, such as whether obesity was covered. There were a considerable number of cases regarding the reasonable accommodation requirement, but this is to be expected given the deliberate flexibility of the concept.

The bulk of the cases regarded procedural issues, which the abbreviated form of the original legislation (in effect one section of an Act, implemented by regulations) rendered necessary. These were issues such as the availability of damages, the ability of individuals to bring actions on their own behalf and whether administrative remedies had to be exhausted first. The detailed ADA has resolved all such issues and built upon the fruits of 15 years of case law under the Rehabilitation Act.

Ideological impact

Chapter 2 emphasised the ideological significance of civil rights laws: their capacity for the empowerment of disabled people and for combating stigma, and dispelling stereotypes, in the broader population. Before examining how the legislation has been applied in practice, I would like to stress the overall impact of these pieces of legislation purely in terms of legislative ideology. The Rehabilitation Act marked a decisive break with the ideological assumptions which had underpinned previous disability laws. Before this Act, the problems experienced by disabled people were understood solely in terms of the individual's own physical or mental limitations, to be remedied by medical means or by providing for their 'special' needs. In contrast, the Rehabilitation Act and ADA address the social and structural constraints which are imposed, and which disable people with impairments.

The Americans with Disabilities Act proclaims the same message but with greatly magnified force. The Rehabilitation Act's anti-discrimination sections were legislative 'afterthoughts', receiving scant legislative or public attention and being incidental to the main purpose of the Act, which focused on the vocational rehabilitation of disabled people. In contrast, the Americans with Disabilities Act proclaims its purpose to be 'to provide a clear and comprehensive mandate for the elimination of discrimination against individuals with disabilities.'[61] It was widely publicised and debated as 'a new bill of rights for the disabled'.[62] This political and social context means that the positive ideological messages contained in embryo in the Rehabilitation Act are magnified and more widely publicised. This is an important development, both because it increases the legislation's capacity for altering public perceptions of the disabled and also because it increases disabled people's awareness of their new rights. Thus, at a practical level, effective enforcement of the Act is more likely.

Both Acts categorise societal exclusion of disabled people as a form of discrimination, particularly the public accommodation provisions of the ADA which powerfully echo the civil rights movement's rejection of segregation. This is tremendously important for disabled people who, as we have seen, have their own history of 'separate but equal' facilities. Most able-bodied people had previously assumed that disabled children and adults were segregated because they could not work or needed special facilities. The Rehabilitation Act (together with the Education of Handicapped Children Act which followed in 1975) made challenging these stereotypes a matter of public policy.

The Rehabilitation Act, and even more so the ADA, contain the seeds of a new public image of disabled people: rights of access presume public participation by disabled people. Bans on job discrimination carry the message that disabled people expect to work, just as requirements of accessibility for colleges and university mean that disabled people pursue higher education. The rights-based concepts of the Rehabilitation Act also provided the framework for a broad alliance with other disadvantaged groups, which was very effectively used in the lobbying for both the Federal Fair Housing Amendment Act 1988 and the ADA itself.

The practical limitations, and continuing stigma, associated with the reasonable accommodation/special needs approach to eliminating structural discrimination admittedly falls short of ideal. However, the tremendous potential for the empowerment of disabled people contained in this legislation far outweighs these limitations. In the period between these two pieces of legislation the American disability movement blossomed in numbers, degree of activism, development of politically sophisticated lobbying and identification as a self-conscious political constituency. At least in part this was in explicit response to the struggle to enforce the Rehabilitation Act. This, in turn, became the crucial factor in the passage of the second, more powerful piece of legislation.

The mobilising capacity of the disability rights movement will determine the scope of the key legal concepts, such as reasonable accommodation and undue hardship, which have been highlighted in this chapter. It will also determine the degree to which the ADA is able to achieve practical change, by ensuring that it is adequately enforced. Ultimately the effectiveness of the ADA can only be predicted by assessing the strengths and nature of the forces which were responsible for passing it. Was it merely passed as 'feel-good' legislation, with no real intention of enforcement? And if it was, can the forces pushing for disability rights prove strong enough to secure effective enforcement? The next chapter will examine these questions, and then look to the record of the Rehabilitation Act as a guide to the potential of the ADA.

4
The Effectiveness of American Laws

This chapter attempts an assessment of American disability discrimination legislation. It discusses the legacy of the Rehabilitation Act 1973 both in its practical outcomes and in so far as it paved the way for the Americans with Disabilities Act 1990 (ADA). Inevitably there is more to say about the impact of the Rehabilitation Act than that of the ADA, but I will also consider the evidence of the impact of the ADA in the short period which has elapsed since it was passed.

This assessment draws on the theoretical considerations outlined previously. One of these concerns the danger of 'reifying' the law, abstracting it from the forces that brought it into being and that will determine the extent to which it is enforced:

> Law is not an act within itself but only the instrument of human actors whose interest it represents. Thus a full consideration of the effects of a particular law cannot be separated from an analysis of the forces that shaped those laws.[1]

Similarly, it would be a mistake to think that the efficacy of a single piece of legislation can be considered without taking into account the broader economic and social conditions that impact powerfully on its ability to produce social change:

> The principle of equality of the law is rightly cherished ... but it is important to understand the narrow limits of this principle. First, however much the legal system may treat individuals and institutions as its equals, it cannot by itself alter the profound inequalities within their actual relationships: law is at best a limited instrument with which to seek greater social justice.[2]

The role of the state in enforcing legislation is particularly crucial in counteracting inequalities between institutions and individuals.

Evaluations of the Rehabilitation Act

How does one evaluate the success of a piece of legislation like the Rehabilitation Act, which is at the same time so broad, covering issues as diverse as higher education, transport and employment, and so restricted in its scope – limited to entities receiving federal grants or contracts?

One important aspect of such an evaluation is the view of intended beneficiaries. A survey by Louis Harris and Associates[3] in 1986 asked 1,000 disabled people if they believed that life had improved for disabled Americans over the last ten years. Seventy per cent believed that life had improved, and two-thirds believed that the federal disability laws had helped a great deal or somewhat. The survey commented that this degree of support for federal laws was unprecedented in the firm's history of surveys.

Higher education

In some areas the achievements of the Rehabilitation Act are readily apparent. Section 504 required colleges and universities to provide programme accessibility and make educational programmes accessible to physically and mentally disabled individuals, as well as to ensure that all new constructions complied with American National Standards Institute specifications for accessibility.

A study jointly conducted by the President's Committee on the Employment of the Handicapped and the American Council for Education shows that in just seven years the numbers of disabled people entering higher education increased threefold, from 2.6 per cent in 1978 to 7.4 per cent in 1985. The report argues that 'such advances would seem to attest to the value of Section 504 of the Rehabilitation Act of 1973 and of other programs which encourage the participation of students with disabilities in higher education.'[4] Whilst the data cannot isolate the sole effects of s. 504, it is clear that it has played a significant role in opening up education opportunities.

Public transport

In other areas the effectiveness of the legislation is more difficult to estimate. The field of public transport was the scene of a tremendous struggle by disabled activists over the interpretation which would be given to the anti-discrimination mandate of s. 504. Public transport was widely affected by the Rehabilitation Act and was the most fiercely contested area, with extensive court battles and street demonstrations. In a sense, the transport provisions of the ADA are as much the product of the processes set in motion by the Rehabilitation Act as the concrete improvements achieved in public transport in the intervening period.[5]

The first set of s. 504 regulations merely required federally supported programmes to make special efforts, but in 1979 the Department of Transportation (DOT) changed course and adopted a requirement of full accessibility, demanding the purchase of accessible buses and the retrofitting of rail mass transit systems. A successful court challenge by the transit industry,[6] contending that the regulations had exceeded statutory authority by imposing 'undue financial burdens' on transit authorities, led in 1981 to a resurrection of the 'special efforts' approach. Responding to pressure from the disability lobby, Congress in 1983 required the DOT to set a new rule establishing minimum service criteria for disabled people. However, it did not require equal access or even comparable services.

The DOT issued service criteria, including a cost cap, to avoid the danger of a renewed challenge from transit authorities on the basis of alleged undue burdens. Transit authorities were not required to spend more than 3 per cent of their operating budgets in satisfying the rules, even if as a consequence they failed to meet the service criteria.

However, it was the disability lobby which succeeded in challenging these regulations through the courts, which decided that this rule was invalid, on the basis that, whilst the DOT was entitled to take costs into account, the strict cost cap was arbitary. In response to this ruling, and in anticipation of the ADA which was progressing through Congress, the DOT announced its intention to draw up rules requiring all new buses to be accessible, and for supplementary paratransit systems to provide a comparable service to that provided to the general public.

Substantial progress has already been made under the Rehabilitation Act, although the nature and level of transport services vary in different localities. Cities like Denver and Seattle are widely regarded as leaders in providing accessible bus services. Nationwide, 35 per cent of the national transit fleet was equipped with accessible features in 1990.[7]

The detailed provisions for both private and public transport were a tremendous achievement for the disabled activists who had struggled to achieve accessible public transport under the Rehabilitation Act. The whole process is vivid testimony to the importance of assessing laws in terms of the social and political forces behind them rather than as documents whose meaning is then deciphered by an impartial court system. These forces will be considered in more detail further on in this chapter.

Employment

Yellin's examination of the Rehabilitation Act's impact on the labour market participation of disabled people is testimony to the importance of an awareness of the constraints which broader economic conditions impose on the effectiveness of legislation.[8] At first glance the statistics summarised by Yellin appear to indicate that the Rehabilitation Act has had no success whatsoever in the area of employment. For example, the average earnings of disabled men as a proportion of those of non-disabled men fell steadily between 1980 and 1988, from 91 to 81 per cent. Yellin, however, places these gloomy labour market indicators within the broader context of labour force trends, and by so doing highlights the limits within which the legislation had to operate. He characterises the position of disabled people in the workforce in the following way: 'Persons with disabilities, like those of minority races, constitute a contingent labour force, suffering displacement first and disproportionately from declining industries and occupations, and experiencing gains only after those without disabilities are no longer available for hire.'[9]

Thus, in the labour force as a whole during these years, the rise in participation amongst young women outstripped the fall in labour force participation amongst older men, although the growth in labour force participation of disabled women was much smaller than the gains of able-bodied women. This in turn was outweighed by the significant drop in the employment of older men with disabilities. The labour force participation of older men with disabilities fell faster than that of those without disabilities. The net result was a 4 per cent drop in the labour force participation of disabled people as a whole.

Yellin argues that the limited success of legislation was due to these broader economic changes in the workforce, and that the Rehabilitation Act was crucial in preventing the impact of these changes having an even worse impact on disabled people's workforce participation. Between 1970 and 1982 the number of government workers grew in absolute terms, and within that the proportion of disabled workers grew from 9.9 per cent to 10.2 per cent. However, from 1982 to 1987 government employment was shrinking, and the percentage of disabled workers fell back from 10.2 per cent to 9.4 per cent. Although the legislation did not succeed in preventing disabled people bearing a disproportionate share of the retrenchment in government employment, Yellin concludes: 'Nevertheless, persons with disabilities [in federal employment] fared much better than those in other sectors of the economy undergoing retrenchment.'[10] He attributes this to the impact of the Rehabilitation Act.

The Equal Employment Opportunity Commission (EEOC) Chairman, Evan Kemp (himself disabled), suggests another significant constraint on the operation of this legislation:

> I don't think employers will notice any dramatic increase in the number of people with disabilities applying for jobs until the early 21st century. For many people with disabilities, marketing themselves will be a completely different way of thinking. Even if they want to work, many will be used to being dependent on welfare. They'll have to wean themselves off dependency before they can develop the self-confidence to go looking for work.[11]

Enforcement of the Rehabilitation Act

Tucker, in her analysis of ten years of enforcement of s. 504 of the Rehabilitation Act, concludes 'while Section 504 has unlocked the door for handicapped persons to enter the mainstream of society, it has failed in its goal of opening the door wide.'[12] She puts forward three reasons for this failure: the limited scope of the law (since remedied by the ADA); conflicting interpretations of the reasonable accommodation requirement (considered in Chapter 3); and the inadequate enforcement of the law. She describes the federal enforcement as 'at best lethargic and at worst ineffectual'.[13]

Procedures

Initially, the procedures for enforcing the anti-discrimination sections of the Rehabilitation Act, and the damages available, were unclear. Complaints under the Act have to be filed with the appropriate government department – the Department of Labor for Section 501, the Office of Federal Contract Compliance Programs (OFCCP) for Section 503, and the relevant federal funding agency for Section 504.

It was initially unclear whether private individuals were also able to bring legal actions in their own right. The Supreme Court eventually established that this was possible for complaints under Section 504, but not the other Sections.[14] District court decisions subsequently established that administrative remedies did not have to be exhausted before individuals were entitled to take legal action. (This is an important point in view of the long delays which were experienced in the government departments' handling of complaints.)

For Sections 501 and 503, no matter how slow the federal investigation, and even in the event of a decision by the administrative agencies not to prosecute, no private right of action is available.

The history of the transport provisions, in which court cases brought by disability groups played a crucial role in extending the scope of s. 504, are eloquent testimony to the importance of empowering the victims of discrimination, by allowing them direct access to courts in their own right. In this way sluggish state enforcement or restrictive interpretations can be challenged and supplemented by individual or group actions.

However, whilst it is essential that individuals are allowed to bring their own court cases, this cannot be a substitute for effective and systematic enforcement on the part of the state. As Tucker observes: 'Most handicapped persons ... do not have the necessary resources to incur the massive expenditures – in terms of both time and money – required to follow a Section 504 action through the courts.'[15] She quotes a legal centre specialising in disability rights: 'Only one in a hundred clients can meet the tests of great facts and law, principle, community and national support, and endurance to get to the filing stage.'[16]

Penalties

The remedies available for Section 503 and 504 violations include reinstatement, or an injunction remedying the discriminatory act, backpay and compensatory damages. Neither punitive nor exemplary damages are available. Contractors risk having their contracts terminated or being debarred from future contracts, whilst funders theoretically risk having their funds withdrawn.

The two factors which are likely to influence organisations to comply with the requirements of the law are the likelihood of penalties being imposed and the scale of risk involved. Effective enforcement increases the risk, whilst high damages awards or the termination of funds and contracts increases the stakes. An article in the *Harvard Business Review* expresses from the employers' perspective what would be required to secure compliance with the law: 'Only damaging court cases and several million dollars of backpay will instil that commitment [to non-discrimination] into employers.'[17]

An example of what can be achieved was a case brought under state anti-discrimination law in Berkeley, California. A jury ordered a restaurant to pay $36,000 compensatory damages, and half a million dollars in punitive damages, to a woman who was barred from access in her wheelchair. Sid Wolinsky, the lawyer from the Disability Rights and Education Fund who took the case, commented: 'There will be a few high profile cases helping business to realize what has to be done. And then, eventually, access for disabled people will become part of the cost of doing business.'[18]

One of the major conflicts which arose during the passage of the ADA was over the issue of whether punitive damages should be available. The extent of the resistance put up by business groups is testimony to the importance of this issue.

The other means of raising the stakes of litigation, which has been used with substantial success in America by women and ethnic minorities, is the class action. A class action is a procedural device by which a group of people with similar interests can sue through a representative of the group, rather than each having to bring a separate case. Class actions have occasionally been brought by disabled litigants. It is not necessary for applicants to share a common disability, provided that they can base their claim on a shared experience of discrimination. In some such cases, brought by a sole employee, a court has made an order benefiting the whole class of persons similarly affected. For example, in *McNutt* v. *Hill*[19] a blind employee of the Department of Housing and Urban Development alleged that the agency's failure to comply with Section 501 had hampered his career.development. The Court required the agency to prepare a report on how it currently met or intended to meet its obligations under the regulations.

By 1980 the opinion of a prominent disabled spokesperson of the federal enforcement record was damning. Frank Bowe very precisely highlights the deficiencies in the implementation process:

The passivity of the Federal role to date in enforcing disability rights is a cause of grave concern. By passivity I mean the administration's failure to move vigorously and visibly to end discrimination on the basis of disability. This failure is evident everywhere: in the over reliance upon individual complaints from disabled persons which penalizes the poorer, the more severely disabled, less politically sophisticated people who may be unaware of their rights; in the dependence upon administrative procedures to the almost total exclusion of tougher measures (funds were rarely cut off even in the face of persistent, blatant violation of the law); in the paucity of appointments for disabled individuals and recognized advocates to leadership positions ... ; in the absence of serious attempts to advise individuals nationwide about their rights; in their chronic under-funding of enforcement activities.[20]

Experience with the enforcement of the Civil Rights Act had already made clear the importance of federal enforcement agencies taking a proactive approach. It was evident that if federal agencies confined themselves to responding to individual complaints their effectiveness would be severely constrained. Not only does such an approach rely on widespread awareness by individuals of their rights and leave complainants vulnerable to retaliation, but it is also inevitably a piecemeal and unsystematic approach. A more strategic enforcement effort is required, with federal agencies responding to individual complaints by bringing their own suits against large employers who are breaking the law, and by cutting off funds and contracts where appropriate.

Chapter 2 has already touched on the importance of affirmative or positive action. Section 501, with regard to federal employers, and Section 503, with regard to federal contractors, both require affirmative action in hiring, placing and promoting disabled people. This entails drawing up plans analysing barriers for disabled people in personnel policies, devising strategies for removing them, and undertaking a systematic outreach programme to recruit more disabled people.

Enforcing contract compliance reviews, with the threat of termination of funds or contracts, and setting quotas for the affirmative action requirements of Sections 501 and 503 would have lent real weight to the anti-discrimination mandate. Joseph Hogan, the chief of the Program Policy branch of the Office of Federal Contract Compliance Programs, was clear about what policies would be effective: 'Our experience has been that to be able to impose and enforce quotas for minorities and women has been immensely helpful ... We would very much be in favor of doing the same thing for disabled people.'[21]

However, in contrast to the position for women and ethnic minorities, the affirmative action requirements of these Sections of the Rehabilitation Act contain no stipulations that contractors or federal employers should set goals or timetables for percentages of disabled employees.

By 1981 it was clear that this approach had failed to have a significant impact and the EEOC introduced a new requirement for federal employers under Section 501. Agencies with more than 500 employees should set numerical goals for the employment of people with targeted disabilities (deafness, 'convulsive disorder', blindness, 'missing extremities', paralysis, mental illness, 'mental retardation' and 'distortion of the limbs or spine').

Clayton Boyd, secretary of the inter-agency committee on disabled employees at the EEOC, argued that such quotas were needed because, despite removing architectural barriers and revising medical standards, the numbers of disabled employees were dropping: 'Quotas put the burden on the employers to identify groups of disabled people who can be brought into the workforce as opposed to leaving it to individuals, discouraged by years of rejection, to come forward.'[22]

Political will

The problems with enforcement stemmed less from ignorance than from a lack of resources within federal enforcement agencies, which in turn reflected a lack of political will. The history of the Rehabilitation Act outlined in Chapter 1 showed how the intervention of disabled activists was necessary to secure the issue of regulations required to implement the Act. Once the Department of Health, Education and Welfare (HEW) had issued its guidelines in 1977, other federal agencies had to issue their own regulations in compliance with these guidelines. By the beginning of 1980 only six agencies had done this, not so much because the issues were seen as complex but because they were accorded low priority and seen as irrelevant to the main goals of agency policy. In 1981 the Paralyzed Veterans of America obtained an injunction requiring the remaining agencies to issue regulations.[23]

Action was also required by the disability movement to secure enforcement of those regulations. Thus in 1977 a court order was obtained forcing HEW to eliminate its backlog of cases promptly and to process all new complaints expeditiously. The order took nearly a year to come into effect because about 1,000 additional members of staff were required to implement it.

Towards the end of Carter's presidency it seemed as though effective enforcement of the Act might commence. The *Harvard Business Review*, for example, published a report with the warning to employers that 'Federal officials are stepping up their efforts to enforce affirmative action requirements.'[24] In one settlement reached by the OFCCP a Texan company was found to have discriminated against 85 employees with a wide range of disabilities based on exclusionary medical standards. The resulting backpay award represented the sort of measure which, if applied more frequently, could have proved effective in altering employers' discriminatory actions.[25]

Political background

However, at precisely the point where progress seemed to be beginning, the Carter administration was replaced by that of Reagan. The new regime was characterised by an emphasis on the deregulation of industry and an intense ideological assault on anti-discriminatory policies, particularly affirmative action. The funding for enforcement agencies was progressively run down. The growth of fiscal conservatism led to the erosion of support for disabled people's civil rights. Opposition by recipient groups intensified, particularly in the crucially important areas of higher education and transport. These struggles are described in some detail by Scotch, Percy and Katzman.[26]

The Reagan administration targeted the Rehabilitation Act regulations as the spearhead of its attempt to 'roll back' federal influence. It was surprised by the strength and political sophistication of the resistance put up by disability rights groups. Groups such as the Disability Rights and Education Fund (DREDEF), a key lobbying and litigation body, had learnt valuable lessons from the struggle to publish the regulations. DREDEF met with key officials in the Department of Justice, which had taken over responsibility for enforcing these sections and for other civil rights groups. It threatened action, both in the courts and in the streets, from a network of groups around the country.

By 1984 the administration was convinced that the disability lobby (for such it now was) was not an easy target. Sensing that the costs were greater than the benefits, the administration abandoned its efforts. However, despite the disability movement's successes in resisting attempts to water down or abolish the regulations, the lack of political will for the enforcement of the legislation took its toll through the starving of funds and resources for enforcement agencies.

Improving the Rehabilitation Act
Ironically, it was this struggle to preserve the regulations which paved the way for the expansion of the anti-discrimination mandate – the Americans with Disabilities Act. In many ways the most staggering thing about the passage of the ADA was that it had the endorsement of a Republican President and the active support of key members of the Republican administration. Cynics have suggested that the charitable, patronising associations of disability made it difficult to oppose a civil rights measure for disabled people. This may hold an element of truth, but the attitude of Republican politicians (and, of course, Democrats also) went beyond passive acquiescence. The disability lobby developed impressive links with the Republican establishment during the process

of defending the Rehabilitation Act regulations. Negotiating sessions first introduced Bush (at that time Vice-President) to Evan Kemp, then head of a Disability Rights Center. Similarly the Attorney-General Dick Thornburgh, who was to prove crucial to the smooth passage of the ADA, developed extensive contacts with DREDEF during this period. The breakthrough for the disability lobby was its success in converting key Republicans to the cause of civil rights for disabled people.

The ADA was the culmination of a steady stream of legal advances for the disabled community. Some of these were defensive, in the sense that they reversed restrictive court interpretations of the Rehabilitation Act. The need to overturn a Supreme Court decision which restricted the reach of both Section 504 and the Civil Rights Act 1964 to programmes directly receiving federal funding (rather than all programmes of an agency in receipt of federal funds) led to the forging of strong links with other civil rights groups.[27] These alliances were to prove vital for the achievement of the ADA, and more immediately led to the passage of the Federal Fair Housing Amendment Act 1988. This Act was largely the result of lobbying by African-American groups for improvements in the enforcement mechanisms in the legislation prohibiting discriminating racism in housing. However, it also extended protection to disabled people for the first time, and thus represents the first federal civil rights measure to link disability discrimination with that faced by other 'minorities'.

It was the President's own National Council on Disability which first proposed a sweeping new federal anti-discrimination law. This Council was converted from an advisory body to the Department of Education into an independent federal agency in 1984, to provide a focus for disability policy. Its 15 members are all appointed by the President.

Congress had requested that the Council review the patchwork of federal laws and programmes affecting disabled people. Its report, *Towards Independence*, recommended 45 legislative improvements, including the first draft of what was to become the ADA.[28] This was favourably received by both Congress and President Reagan. In 1988 a follow-up report was produced, containing a draft Bill.[29] Immediately afterward Bills modelled on this draft were introduced in both the Senate and the House of Representatives, attracting considerable support.

It would, however, be a mistake to conclude that this initiative was a paternalist gesture, initiated by the establishment in the same manner as the Rehabilitation Act. On the contrary, the initiative, and the broad political support which it quickly received, was testimony to the success of the disability movement's lobbying and increasing political clout. A quote from a disgruntled opponent is probably the most eloquent witness to the impact of this lobbying:

The White House rushed to strike a deal with Senator Edward Kennedy and the disability lobbyists. The White House Director of policy developments, Bill Roper, helped Senate Labor Committee staffer Robert Silverstein and disability lobbyists draft the compromise Bill. Ever since, the Administration has refused to deviate from the disability and civil rights lobbies' position. Republican staffers say that all amendments were referred by the Administration to Pat Wright, Executive Director of DREDEF. Ms Wright and Chai Feldblum, legislative counsel for the American Civil Liberties Union, not only helped write the Bill, they called most of the shots throughout the legislative process.[30]

Nevertheless, some compromises were necessary to secure the passage of the Bill. The modification requirements for public accommodations and employment were watered down. In the original draft such modifications would have been required unless they could be shown to 'fundamentally alter or threaten the existence' of the business or facility. The compromise Bill only required 'readily achievable' modifications to public accommodations, and employment accommodations which did not cause 'undue hardship'. Other compromises were over restricting damages in public accommodations cases and longer phasing in periods for the provisions of the Act to take effect. There was also some reduction in the scope of the Bill. Originally almost all businesses open to the public were covered, but the list of those covered is still significantly broader than the coverage of the Civil Rights Act 1964. The final heated debate, won by the disability lobby without compromise, was over the right-wing proposal that people with Aids, the 'non-deserving', unacceptable face of disability, should be excluded from coverage.

After the defeat of this proposal, the compromise Bill, having been endorsed by both presidential candidates, was reintroduced in 1989 and achieved a swift and trouble-free passage.

As we have seen, the contacts forged by disability activists with key members of the Republican administration when resisting regulatory cut-backs proved crucial in achieving the ADA. But precisely how did they persuade a naturally conservative, laissez-faire administration? Evan Kemp, the Republican Commissioner for the EEOC, predicted in 1988 that a disability rights Bill applying to private organisations would soon be passed. His reasons are revealing. He argued that 'disabled people and the parents of disabled people were simply too numerous and too politically active for this not to happen'.[31] Tony Coelho, a Democratic Congressman who was one of the chief sponsors of the bill, echoed this sentiment: 'Disability impacts practically every family.'[32]

Indeed, it is interesting to note the connections with disability of many of the politicians closely associated with the Bill. Edward Kennedy has a sister with learning difficulties and a son who lost a leg to cancer; Senator Weicker has a child with Down's Syndrome; Senator Bob Dole has a paralysed right arm; and the chief Senate sponsor, Tim Harkin, has a deaf brother and paralysed nephew. The Attorney-General, Dick Thornburgh, whose support was crucial to the success of the Bill, has a son with learning difficulties, while former President Bush has two sons with disabilities.

The critical factor was that these politicians now identified themselves or their family members as disabled, rather than hiding this attribute through shame. Millions of voters went through the same process of identification as a result of the activities of the disability movement. The new class consciousness of disabled people was revealed in a 1986 poll in which 74 per cent said they felt a common identity with other disabled people.[33] In this respect the Voting Accessibility for the Elderly and Handicapped Act 1984 had not only the practical significance of ensuring that disabled people were able to vote, but also had a tremendous symbolic significance, marking the recognition of disabled people as a political constituency.

The essential underpinning of these increasingly successful lobbying activities was the grass-roots militancy of the disability movement. This contributed to securing strategic victories and also to the broader process of altering public opinion. The activities of the Aids movement, ACT-UP, are probably the best known of these struggles, and the Aids lobby was a powerful ally in the achievement of ADA.

The deaf community also made a significant contribution, with the student uprising at Gallaudet University, in particular, securing world-wide publicity for their struggles. Gallaudet University is the world's only liberal arts university specifically for deaf people. In 1988 the Board of Trustees elected a hearing person as its president. The ensuing protest of both students and staff succeeded after a week in changing the appointment to that of the first deaf president in Gallaudet's history. The impact of this struggle reached far beyond the immediate issues, as deaf people used the media attention to promote an awareness of their culture and language, and to demand that they should control their own affairs. A new sensitivity to the needs of deaf people was apparent in a spate of Bills through Congress and in the telecommunications provisions of the ADA.[34]

The disability movement was able to capitalise on this political leverage by astute lobbying, pitching the message in terms calculated to appeal to the Republicans. They emphasised the reduction of welfare expenditure and meeting the needs of business. In doing so they were able to build on the changing demographics of disability. The ageing of the population in particular has contributed to the growth in the numbers of disabled people. By 1990 there were 6.2 million elderly Americans with one or more disabilities, an increase from 5 million in 1984. This both boosted the lobby power described above and meant that disabled people could be pointed to as an important market and social constituency.

Enforcing the ADA

As with the Rehabilitation Act, federal enforcement agencies have been given responsibility for publicising the ADA, issuing regulations, dealing with complaints, conducting strategic investigations and, where appropriate, initiating litigation. The agency with responsibility for enforcing the employment provisions is the EEOC. The Department of Justice has responsibility for the public services and accommodation sections (Titles II and III), whilst the DOT and the Federal Communications Commission respectively have responsibility for enforcing the transport and telecommunication requirements (Titles II:ii and IV). Unlike the position under the earlier Act, it is clearly established that individuals can take legal proceedings on their own behalf, without relying on these federal agencies.

The remedies available are also more substantial than they were under the preceding Act. One of the key struggles during the passage of the Bill was over the disability lobby's demand that damages should be in line with those available to victims of sex and race discrimination under the Civil Rights Act 1964. This would have meant that whilst backpay, injunctions, reinstatement and lawyers' fees could be awarded, punitive damages could not. (These are damages over and above those which a court thinks necessary to compensate a victim, designed to punish perpetrators and act as a deterrent.)

The issue was complicated by the simultaneous attempts by civil rights groups to amend the Civil Rights Act to enable precisely such punitive damages to be awarded in cases of sex and race discrimination. The administration attempted to pass an amendment to the ADA to ensure that in the event of civil rights groups succeeding, punitive damages would still not be awarded for disability discrimination. This amendment was defeated by disability lobbyists arguing that it would perpetuate discrimination against disabled people by putting them in an inferior position to other minority groups.

When the Civil Rights Restoration Act 1991 was eventually passed, compensatory (that is, damages to compensate for the full economic loss, as well as the pain suffered by victims of discrimination) and punitive damages became available for cases of intentional employment discrimination under the ADA. Damages can be awarded by juries, which tends to increase the amounts awarded. In public accommodation cases, however, there are no jury trials and no damages are available to individual litigants. What the courts can do is issue injunctions forcing businesses to remove barriers, and award lawyers' fees. In addition, damages up to $50,000 for a first offence and $100,000 for subsequent offences can be awarded where cases are brought by the Attorney-

General. S/he has the duty of investigating alleged violations of the public accommodation provisions, including periodic compliance reviews. S/he is empowered to take legal action if s/he has 'reasonable cause' to believe that any person or group of persons is engaged in a 'pattern or practice'[35] of discrimination, or where s/he believes that discrimination has occurred which raises a point of public importance.

These penalties should prove sufficiently strong to encourage voluntary compliance with the ADA provisions, and to provide adequate recompense to encourage individuals to take legal action where such compliance has not been achieved. They represent a significant achievement for the disability lobby.

The problems which are likely to arise stem not so much from inadequate enforcement mechanisms or remedies, but from the lack of adequate resources for enforcement. One leading disabled activist takes a jaundiced view of the new Act:

> Regrettably, disabled people are not sufficiently organized to press for the kind of enforcement that would make ADA more than a public spirited gesture, and the Bush Administration knows it. That is why it can afford to back the measure.[36]

The change to a Democratic President in 1993 may augur well for future enforcement. Certainly Clinton has made some high-profile appointments of disabled activists, such as Judy Heuman. However, the initial reports of the implementation process all echo this concern about enforcement resources. The first, and often lengthiest, stage in implementing a law is publicising it. A Gallup poll in 1991 indicated that much work remains to be done in this area; it showed that 42 per cent of businesses were unfamiliar with the requirements of the ADA.[37]

Victoria Scott's *Lessons from America*, the first published attempt in Britain at a preliminary assessment of the impact of the ADA, reports encouraging progress, but stresses the need for more resources for both information and enforcement activities.[38] She says that although some federal provision has been made, more information is required about what assistive technology is available to comply with the law's requirements, as well as general advice about how to achieve compliance cost effectively.

The delays which Scott reports in federal agencies resolving individual complaints seem to parallel the enforcement problems experienced with the Rehabilitation Act. However, because the essential groundwork for the ADA has been better prepared, at least some of those earlier problems will be avoided. Thus the regulations for the ADA, in striking contrast to those of the Rehabilitation Act, were all issued within a year of the passage of the Act, after wide public consultation. The early years of enforcement of the Rehabilitation Act were hampered by doubts about the rights of individuals to take up cases and the damages which were available, whilst with the ADA both of these issues have been favourably resolved.

The United States General Accounting Office commissioned an evaluation to examine whether access for disabled people to public and private services had improved since the passage of the ADA.[39] In January 1992, 231 randomly selected businesses and government facilities were visited by a team assessing their accessibility. At the same time people with mobility and sensory impairments were surveyed to discover how often and where they had found access barriers in the previous six months. The research team visited those places likely to have more barriers for people with disabilities (older cities in states with less protective laws). They concluded that most features of businesses and government facilities were accessible to disabled people but that a number of important barriers remained. They highlighted the need for continuing educational activities and technical assistance, since many businesses were unclear about their legal obligations or how best to achieve barrier removal.

The Gallup poll mentioned above found that 33 per cent of the businesses surveyed had removed barriers in the period between the passage of the ADA and its commencement date.[40]

The National Council on Disability reported on the progress of the ADA one year after its provisions had come into effect.[41] The research team surveyed organizations representing the disability community and those covered by the ADA (businesses and local government) as well as federal enforcement agencies, and used media sources, public hearings, a toll-free telephone line and other correspondence from concerned parties. It came to broadly the same conclusions as those of the other studies: that significant progress had been made despite the need for a greater awareness of the law. Given the short time frame since implementation had begun, they concluded: 'The most remarkable observation about these beginnings is that so much has been achieved in so little time ... Witnesses at ADA Watch hearings from organizations representing covered entities portrayed a very favorable picture of the efforts of business, state and local governments and other covered entities to implement the ADA.'[42]

The council noted the need for caution in interpreting these reports and, in common with the other reports, stressed the need for more resources for information and technical assistance, as well as substantial research on the progress and impact of the ADA: 'These reports of significant progress must be viewed cautiously because they only represent those organizations with an awareness of the ADA ... ADA implementation has been greatly hindered by lack of information and technical assistance.'[43]

The report contains interesting data about the nature of complaints under the new law. In the first six months after ADA provisions came into effect the Department of Justice received 450 complaints about state services and public accommodations. In the first six months after the employment provisions commenced, the EEOC received 4,299 charges of discrimination. Almost half of these related to dismissal, and a further 20 per cent to requirements for reasonable accommodation.

The report also lists ADA related cases, such as a reporter who uses a wheelchair, bought a ticket for a show but was unable to attend when ushers refused to help him up the flight of seven steps, and a law graduate who sued the Connecticut Bar Examining Committee when it insisted that he answer questions about mental illness on the application form. Many examples were also provided of pre-emptive compliance actions.

After the first year of enforcing the employment provisions the EEOC issued a summary of achievements.[44] It had handled over 11,000 complaints on disability discrimination, about 15 per cent of its overall workload on enforcing civil rights statutes. Over 2,000 had been resolved, with compensation granted to claimants amounting to over $11 million. The EEOC had filed two ADA law suits in court. The first was on behalf of the Executive Director of a security company who had been forced to retire on being diagnosed as having brain cancer. The EEOC alleged that he was capable of doing his job, and was fired illegally. He was awarded $222,000. The other case involved the lower benefits paid out for Aids under a workplace medical plan.

Scott lays particular emphasis on the visible increase in social participation by disabled people, and the powerful impact which this has in challenging stereotypes:

> The ADA has also had an impact on the visibility of disabled people within society which is a useful indication of improved integration. Not only in shops and restaurants, but on TV programmes, in movies and advertisements, old stereotypical roles are being disregarded in favour of positive images. This in itself plays a major part in increasing public awareness of disabled people's experiences, which facilitates the further integration of disabled people into mainstream society.[45]

Many other accounts convey vividly, albeit impressionistically, the wide-reaching transformations which these disability laws have achieved in American society, penetrating everyday life in a myriad small but crucial ways:

> Braille dots are popping up next to numbers on automatic teller machines. Phones for the deaf are being established in sports arenas ... From offices to movie theaters, the impact of the most sweeping

piece of civil rights legislation ever enacted is being seen, heard and felt ... When Congress passed the law designed to open jobs and access to the nation's 43 million disabled people, business angrily warned it would drive companies into bankruptcy and clog the courts with lawsuits ... but the predicted battles haven't materialised.[46]

Ultimately the implementation of the Act will be determined by the capacity of the disability movement to push for effective enforcement and for the broadest possible interpretation of the legislative mandate. The resounding recognition represented by the ADA of the centrality of discrimination in the lives of disabled people, and its endorsement of the need for structural alterations in society, will serve to boost the self-confidence of disabled people and counter the stereotypes of dependency and incapacity still prevalent in the wider population.

At the same time the success of the Act in achieving the profound social changes which are necessary to end the subordination of disabled people will, at least in part, depend on broader political factors, such as the degree of commitment to civil rights generally and to social provisions such as education and health. The state of the economy is also likely to be of crucial importance, as is the extent to which potential opponents, such as business interests, can be convinced that it is in their interests to include disabled people as clients and employees.

Amidst all the celebrations surrounding the passage of the ADA a leading disability activist sounded a warning note: 'One of the best ways to kill a civil rights concept is to pass a law and not enforce it.'[47] However, as long as the civil rights movement of disabled people is alive and kicking the ADA provides an immensely valuable weapon for pushing for the proclaimed goals of equality, integration and full participation.

Without action no good

5
Importing Anti-discrimination Laws

When considering the effect of anti-discrimination legislation in Britain, account must be taken of the differences between Britain and the United States in terms of constitutional and legal frameworks, and political, cultural and legal traditions. These enormous differences have a determining effect on how the laws operate in practice.

Chapter 6 will examine the experience of the earlier imports relating to sex and race discrimination, to see if there are lessons which could usefully be drawn upon in terms of 'importing' disability rights. First, however, this chapter takes a broader look at the different soil into which, if the disability movement has its way, disability rights laws will be transplanted. It examines the political role of the law in the two countries, and in particular their histories with regard to rights and equality issues.

The most immediate explanation for the different roles played by the law in the politics of the two countries lies in their constitutional systems. Unlike Britain, America has a written constitution and the American Supreme Court acts as its guardian, with the power to overturn acts of either the legislative or the executive arms of the body politic. Holland, in his comparative study of judicial activism, emphasises that the constitutional role of the Supreme Court is an explicitly political one, stemming from its role as guarantor of a written constitution and Bill of Rights.[1] He quotes de Tocqueville: 'Scarcely any political question arises in the United States that is not resolved sooner or later into a judicial question.'[2]

This constitutional jurisdiction legitimates judicial policy making. 'The Supreme Court stands too at the interface between legal and political process, a fact of which both public and judiciary are very conscious.'[3] Politics is accepted as the proper sphere for law, and conversely law is accepted as political. Federal judges are appointed by the President, whilst state judges are either appointed by politicians or elected. They are accustomed to being seen as political actors.

Holland contrasts the situation in Britain, where the system, based on an unwritten constitution and parliamentary sovereignty, is the major barrier to judicial activism. In the absence of a written constitution Parliament has unfettered power to legislate on any subject and no other body has the power to challenge the legitimacy of Acts of Parliament.

However, the entry of Britain into the European Economic Community (which subsequently became the European Community, or EC) in 1973 has introduced fundamental change into this situation. In matters over which the EC has jurisdiction, British laws and their interpretation by the judiciary can be challenged in the European Court of Justice. We will see in Chapter 6 that this has had particular impact in the area of discrimination law.

In Britain, the actions of executive agencies can only be reviewed by the judiciary on very restricted grounds. They can be challenged on the basis that they are ultra vires (outside the legal powers of the agencies); that there has been a breach of procedural correctness; or that the actions are 'unreasonable'. The last has a very narrow scope: decisions may only be overturned on the basis that no rational person could possibly have reached that conclusion.[4]

This is in no way intended to imply that British judges have no role in policy making. It is not an overt role, however, and the screen of judicial impartiality enables a politically unaccountable judiciary to maintain a fiercely conservative tradition. Professor Griffith has given the best-known critique of the myths of judicial impartiality and political neutrality in his book, *The Politics of the Judiciary*:

> My thesis is that judges in the United Kingdom cannot be politically neutral because they are placed in positions where they are required to make political choices which are sometimes presented to them, and often presented by them, as determinations of where the public interest lies; that their interpretation of what is in the public interest and therefore desirable is determined by the kind of people they are.[5]

Discrimination in British law

The main focus of Griffith's book is on the industrial relations record of the judiciary, particularly during the industrial strife of the 1970s. However, he also discusses its role in human rights issues, and concludes that the dominant approach of the courts has been to regard the issue of discriminatory treatment as of little importance, either in terms of individual rights or of the 'public interest'. The judiciary has tended to proceed on the basis that anti-discrimination legislation interferes with the freedom of individuals to discriminate, and the public interest is therefore best served by restricting the impact of that legislation to the maximum extent, thus implicitly valuing the freedom of discriminators above the rights of individuals to be free from discriminatory treatment.

Lester and Bindman's study focuses specifically on the history of judicial treatment of racial discrimination.[6] They conclude that the reluctance on the part of the British judiciary to acknowledge its public policy role leads to a constricting formalism, which fatally narrows the scope of judicial interpretation by treating legal issues as 'linguistic problems to be solved in a moral vacuum'.[7]

Focusing purely on the technicalities of the law has left the specific interpretation in individual cases at the mercy of the prejudices of individual judges, since arguments can usually be conjured up on both sides. Lester and Bindman argue that: 'Judicial failure to develop an explicit sense of public policy, instead of preserving certainty and predictability in the law, sometimes had the opposite effect.'[8] Their review of cases up to the Race Relations Act 1968 reveals that where judges wished to deny effect to legal actions they were capable of very creative use of technicalities. Perhaps the thinnest excuse for judical prejudice is found in the judgement in *De Costa* v. *Paz*.[9] The case involved a bequest for the propagation of the Jewish faith. At a time when bequests for the promotion of Christianity were regular occurrences, this Jewish bequest was held to be void on the basis that it was for a superstitious purpose.

Although judges have the power to set aside or refuse to enforce contracts on the basis that they are contrary to public policy or morality (as with the Jewish bequest), they have declined to use this power where discrimination is the issue. There has been no judicial ruling that acts of racial discrimination committed in Britain are contrary to public policy. This approach, by disregarding the issue of racial hatred, conveys the message that such motivation is therefore acceptable in public policy terms.

One example cited by Lester and Bindman is a 1931 Privy Council case[10] involving a Kenyan Asian. The court ruled that the colonial Commissioner of Lands was entitled to use his official powers to prevent non-whites from purchasing land in certain areas. In classic British manner, the judges purported to avoid the ethical and social implications of their decision by merely applying 'legal reasoning', examining the powers of the Commissioner rather than the purposes for which they were applied. Just as the Commissioner had the power to restrict the sale of land for particular purposes by particular people, so he could restrict the sale to particular racial groups. Lester and Bindman make explicit the value judgement hidden behind this veil of neutrality: 'The judges were, half-consciously perhaps, making a value judgement that racial restrictions had as rational and legitimate a basis as commercial restrictions.'[11]

The case of Nagle provided a rare glimpse of the potential which the British law could have, notwithstanding its constitutional restrictions, to curb discrimination.[12] Miss Nagle was a horse trainer, who complained that the Jockey Club had refused her a trainer's licence purely on the basis of her gender, and that this practice was contrary to public policy.

The Court of Appeal looked favourably on her claim. Lord Denning stated as a principle of public law that a person has a right to work at his or her profession, 'without being unjustly excluded from it at the whim of those having governance of it'.[13] Arbitrary or unreasonable exclusions were 'against public policy',[14] and the courts would not give them effect. Lord Justice Danckwerts declared that 'the law relating to public policy cannot remain immutable. It must change with the passage of time.'[15]

This ruling, however, was confined to monopoly situations, and is significant not so much as an example of progressive tendencies within the courts, since it remains an isolated example, but as an indication of the creative approach which would have been open to other courts, if they had chosen to follow it. On the vast majority of occasions they have declined to do so. Where judges have overturned discriminatory restrictions it has tended to be on technical, legal terms rather than on grounds of public policy:

> English judges tend to treat equality before the law ... as a formal concept concerning equal access to the courts, legal procedures and remedies, not as a principle which entitles them ... to restrain a stronger party from oppressing a weaker one.[16]

It was the absence of judicial responsiveness to racial (and sexual) injustices which necessitated the passage of the sex and race statutes in the 1970s. In the United States, on the contrary, a stream of Supreme Court decisions from the early 1950s onwards furthered legal protection against racial discrimination, and preceded the passage of the key equality statute, the Civil Rights Act 1964, which extended the constitutional principle of equality into the private sphere.[17]

Discrimination in American law

In America, the Fourteenth Amendment to the constitution proclaims the principle that 'equal protection of the laws' shall be afforded to all persons. The power of this legal principle stems from its political roots and resonance. It was passed after a bloody civil war, the key issue in which came to be seen as the abolition of slavery and its associated features. This is not to say that this principle of equal treatment of races by the state has not proved capable of distortion precisely because of changes in the prevailing politics of race. A series of Supreme Court cases in the early 1870s distorted the purpose of the Civil War Amendments, most notably through a ruling that the Fourteenth Amendment did not prevent legal segregation, provide it was 'equal'.[18]

These cases reflected a tidal shift in American politics – the political compromise between Northern industrialists and the white Southern ruling class that brought to an end the 'Reconstruction' period during which attempts were made to incorporate black Southerners into the economy and polity on terms of some equality.[19] The point is not that the American constitution provides principles of protection for citizens which override political shifts, but rather the opposite – there is a more explicit recognition that these decisions are political ones, and that issues of race are of central importance to American politics.

Clearly this politicisation of judicial decision-making has its own dangers. But these may be less significant than the creeping evasion and covert support for the status quo of the British judiciary. Moreover, Supreme Court constitutional decisions are not mere reflections of the current administration's politics. Despite the fact that they are presidential appointments, the personnel of the courts hold office for life. Supreme Court epochs are therefore frequently out of step with current electoral politics, providing either a check (as when it thwarted a series of New Deal measures under Roosevelt) or a source of change (as during the 1950s and 1960s, principally on the subject of race discrimination).

Disability in the constitution

The Fourteenth Amendment has been interpreted as providing differing levels of protection to different groups. This is expressed through the varying constitutional standards of scrutiny which are applied to legislation: a 'strict' standard for distinctions based on race,[20] and an 'intermediate' standard for women.[21]

On the basic issue of disabled people's right to protection against discriminatory treatment by the state, the constitutional law has not been helpful. The issue was not decided until the case of *Cleburne Living Center* in 1985, by which time the statutory law had already expanded protection against discrimination to disabled people. Moreover, although a level of constitutional protection was established by this case, it has not been successfully invoked since. The Supreme Court refused to regard disability as a 'suspect classification' (which in constitutional law triggers heightened levels of scrutiny by the courts). Therefore, provided state actions which discriminate against disabled people are rationally related to a legitimate government objective, they cannot be challenged under the constitution.[22] Constitutional principles have therefore been of limited value in furthering the rights of disabled people. They have been most fruitful in the area of education[23] and in providing mentally ill people with a degree of protection from abuse.[24] In both of these fields lobbying groups developed a legal strategy which not only established the existence of constitutional protections, but also fed into a broader political campaign, successfully raising the importance of the issues.

Nevertheless, the indirect impact of the constitutional position has been of incalculable value. The broader acceptance by judges that their decisions should take into account public policy issues, and that the principle of equal treatment was a key public goal, has had an immeasurably progressive impact on their interpretation of statutory law.

The constitutional position has had a similar impact on the ability of lawyers to make use of the courts as part of a political strategy. Just as the civil disobedience tactics of the civil rights movement influenced those of the disability movement, so have the legal strategies of the Legal Defence Fund of the National Association for the Advancement of Colored People (NAACP) served as a model for the strategic use of the court system. Consequently, legal strategies played a crucial role both in the development of American disability rights statutes, and in the struggle to achieve their implementation:

> An ... important factor in the development of Section 504 was the expanding case law involving the rights of disabled people. While this legal trend did not play a direct role in the initial drafting of the statute, it did provide a philosophical and conceptual basis for much of the regulation and for subsequent litigation.[25]

Procedural differences

The acknowlegement by American courts that their decisions will have public policy implications, and the acceptance that these should properly be taken into account when reaching those decisions, has had significant impact on legal procedures. American tools such as class actions, amicus briefs and brandeis briefs have been developed to enable the broader implications of decisions to be fairly considered, and thereby to reduce the individual focus inherent in the Western legal system.

Class actions are not generally possible in British courts, which insist on separate cases being brought by all individual members of the affected group. Not only is this much more expensive and time-consuming, but a class action enables a more authoritative resolution of an issue.

Another useful procedural device is the amicus brief. This is a legal submission to the court, presented not by a party to the case but by an amicus curiae – an interested party giving assistance to the court. The presentation of such briefs is common in America, and enables the group consequences of litigation to be identified.

A brandeis brief allows the admission of sociological and other contextual material not normally admissible under the laws of evidence. This device facilitates the bolder line on policy making taken by American courts, allowing greater socio-legal analysis.[26] Census statistics, official research and reports, and the work of experts in law, history and social sciences have all been used, for example, to help establish cases of indirect discrimination.

A further factor which lessens the individual focus of court proceedings is the absence of the British concept of 'mootness'. Generally only persons who are directly affected by a decision in a way which the court considers sufficient can challenge it. One of the restrictions that this imposes is that authorities will frequently settle individual test cases to head off unfavourable precedents. Lawyers must accept on the individual's behalf, as it is in their client's best interest, but in Britain this means that it is no longer possible to continue the litigation. In America, the Supreme Court has accepted a much more flexible approach to the mootness principle. A legal challenge will not be thwarted by intervening acts of a party to the case.

Legal lobbying

Every bit as significant as these increased procedural flexibilities in the American system are the divergences in the attitudes of the public to the law, and in particular the extent to which it is seen as a political resource. Holland claims that the United States is 'the most litigious country in the world',[27] and attributes the 'rights consciousness' of Americans to the prominent role which the judiciary plays in policy formation.

Certainly Americans have a stronger sense of the importance of the role of the law as an instrument of policy making. The massive media attention focused on the selection of Supreme Court justices is testimony to the significance attached to their role. In Britain, in comparison, even people with considerable interest and involvement in public affairs are unlikely to be able to name a single member of the highest court, the Law Lords.

In America, public awareness has been fed by the use of the law by political activists, particularly civil rights groups like the NAACP. Although there is a long history of pressure groups in America using the law as a resource in their campaigns, the 1960s and 1970s in particular witnessed an explosion of public interest law groups, both on the left and the right. Funding sources played a significant role in this development. For example, the Legal Services Program of the Office of Equal Opportunity set up in 1965 assisted this trend by providing funding for collective action at a local level.

When looking at the different roles that legal campaigning has played it is wise to look beyond the legal sphere, to the broader differences in the political structures of the two countries. In part the greater strength of legal lobbying groups in America reflects their strength generally, and their importance in the political system. A report by Richard Scotch on the situation with regard to disability politics in Britain emphasises this point:

In comparing the strength of advocacy organisations working on behalf of disabled people in the United States and Great Britain, it is important to understand the differences in political and social institutions between the two nations. British society contains a number of implicit but powerful traditions which surround government policies, making it difficult for reformers to alter established relationships and institutions without the full strength of the government behind them.[28]

In recent years the US party system has weakened and individual legislators have gained more autonomy. American parties are loose coalitions of interest groups, in contrast to the continuing class-based nature of British parties, and are much less controlled by their leaders than is the case in Britain.[29] This leaves them much more accessible to approaches by lobbying groups representing particular interests:

It is widely accepted by political scientists that support for traditional political parties declined during the 1960s to be replaced by a new loyalty towards the idea of 'cause' or 'single issue' groups. Whatever the reason ... there has been an explosion in American pressure and interest groups since the Second World War and the increase has escalated since 1975.[30]

Above all, the critical influence of the civil rights movement in inspiring and providing models for other minority groups seeking to secure equal participation in society cannot be overemphasised. In the words of Scotch, 'It provided the models through popular actions in support of equal rights, statutory language protecting those rights, and administrative structures for formulating formal procedures.'[31] Whilst the American civil rights movement has also had an impact in Britain, and has provided inspiration for protest movements there, inevitably this influence is weaker.

In general, the influence of lobby groups or even social movements is weaker in Britain than in America. A major reason for this is that the British parliamentary system is much more 'majoritarian' than the American system, and majority party status is seldom affected by 'peripheral' issues such as disability. In Britain the ability to shape policy depends more on influencing the positions and priorities of the political parties.

Britain changes?

The British legal profession has historically been more wary of the taint of political involvement than its American counterpart has. Harlow and Rawlings suggest that as a result of ingrained traditions, 'Lawyers are quick to divest their case law of its political and social significance, reducing it to a boxed set of sanitised legal precedents'.[32]

Harlow and Rawlings set out to compare legal lobbying in Britain and America, and in the process disclosed a hitherto unrecognised British history of pressure group litigation.[33] Their study shows that in recent years there has been a significant growth in public interest law and in its use as a tool to secure political changes. The Child Poverty Action Group (CPAG), for example, has shifted from a 'Fabian' style of lobbying, presenting information to key figures in Westminster and Whitehall, to one which incorporates the use of legal test cases[34] and MIND, the leading mental health interest group, turned in the 1970s to an increasing emphasis on rights enforcement.[35]

Cooper[36] largely attributes these changes to the surrounding politics of the period. The process was heralded by the law centre movement, reflecting the local community-based activism of the 1970s. The general growth in pressure groups and social movements clearly contributed to the increasing resort to legal strategies. Paradoxically the Thatcher period of radical conservatism, with the government's distaste for parliamentary accountability, also fuelled the process. Lobby groups that were no longer able to focus on insider dealing turned to the courts instead. 'In the era of conviction politics and domination by one political party of political institutions, courts are increasingly asked to assume the function of a surrogate political process.'[37]

Holland notes a corresponding trend, beginning in the 1970s, for increasing judicial activism.[38] Most prominently in the case of Lord Denning, judges have proved themselves increasingly, if sometimes reluctantly, ready to make public policy in contentious areas. The Gillick case, involving the issue of contraceptive advice for an under-age teenager, is perhaps the most obvious example of such cases.[39]

Perhaps the most visible change in the legal politics of rights is the increasing popularity of proposals for a Bill of Rights.[40] A discussion of the arguments for and against this proposal would fill a book in itself. Whilst there is little chance of achieving this goal in the short term, if ever, the debate itself is symptomatic of the broader changes in the political and legal culture around rights issues.

Changes in the legal system

The increase in the use of public law as a political tool has produced some loosening up of procedural techniques. However, it is wise to keep these changes in perspective. Holland concludes his study of judicial activism: 'Measured by the standards of other Anglo-American democracies, English activism hardly even approaches a threshold that might bear that name.'[41]

Changes in the use of law have also both provoked and reflected changes within the legal profession itself. Harlow and Rawlings suggest that: 'Slowly the legal profession is becoming less homogeneous ... This in turn is creating a pool of lawyers sympathetic to pressure through law.'[42] They claim that this in turn has produced changes in the legal culture and ethos. It would be foolish, however, to overlook the resistance of the legal profession to opening up to new groups. The Society of Black Lawyers has been particularly active in scrutinising the discriminatory practices which serve to retain the white exclusivity of the legal world. A committee of enquiry set up by the Bar Council concluded in its interim report that black students suffered indirect discrimination at the Council for Legal Education.[43]

The Race Relations Committee of the Law Society has similarly challenged the procedures for the selection of judges, on the same basis of indirect discrimination. In an article for the *New Law Journal*, Geoffrey Bindman has examined the possible basis for such a claim.[44] He notes that in 1991, whilst 6 per cent of the practising bar were black, there were no black judges in the House of Lords, Court of Appeal or High Court, and only two out of 447 circuit judges were black. The Lord Chancellor is responsible for all judicial appointments (including members of tribunals), acting upon the recommendations of senior judges, according to criteria labelled by Bindman as 'nebulous'. The Lord Chancellor describes the criteria for selection as: 'considered by unidentified judges to have appropriate professional ability, experience, standing, integrity, a sound temperament and the physical ability to carry out the duties of the office'.[45]

Bindman points to a finding by a Commission for Racial Equality (CRE) investigation[46] that 'word of mouth' recruitment by recommendation of members of an all-white workforce amounted to unlawful discrimination. The Code of Practice,[47] approved by the Secretary of State for Employment, suggests that employers should not recruit through the recommendations of existing employees where the workforce is wholly or predominantly white.

In so far as these practices strengthen the operation of the old boy network they also have adverse effects on women. (At the time of Bindman's article, whilst 18 per cent of practising barristers were women only 6 per cent of assistant recorders, the lowest rung of the judiciary, were women, and the proportion of women sharply declined in the higher ranks.)

Chapter 1 quoted a survey of disabled solicitors showing the impact of prejudice and physical access barriers on their careers. The same factors restrict the appointment of disabled judges, jurists and magistrates. Back in 1982 the Committee on Restrictions against Disabled People (CORAD) report highlighted this problem (for the background to this report, see Chapter 8)

A lady in a wheelchair was called for jury service at the Crown Court. She telephoned the Clerk to ascertain the position regarding access, but was told that on no account could they consider having a wheelchair in court; subsequently, against her wishes, she was exempted from jury service for life.[48]

Blind and deaf people have been exempted from jury service on the basis that as they cannot see or hear the defendant they cannot therefore assess his or her guilt. It has also been suggested that the presence of visibly disabled people on the jury would undermine the public's confidence in the judicial system. Chapter 6 will consider the likely impact that this bias towards able-bodied, white males in the judiciary has on the quality of justice which they provide to the community as a whole.

This chapter has suggested a number of ways in which rights-based laws may be easier to pass, and more likely to take effect, in America than in Britain. This is not intended to suggest that such laws cannot be introduced and made effective in the latter country, but rather to draw attention to the additional obstacles which need to be tackled. The development of lobby groups and the politicisation of law and lawyers are factors which suggest that these barriers may not be insurmountable. Britain also has a tremendous advantage in being able to use the American experience as a guide to what is possible, and to learn from their achievements.

6
British Race and Sex Laws – Could Do Better

Any British legislation protecting disabled people against discrimination will inevitably be modelled on existing sex and race legislation. Clearly, this model will need to be adapted to the particular issues presented by disability discrimination, and Chapter 7 will consider these in the British context. First, however, this chapter considers the difficulties experienced in implementing the sex and race discrimination laws, together with the extent to which the structural framework of these is deficient, and should be revised for any new disability rights law.

Four Acts set out the law with regard to sex and race discrimination: the Equal Pay Act 1970 applies to discriminatory pay differentials between men and women, whilst the Sex Discrimination Act 1975 covers all other aspects of gender discrimination. The Sex Discrimination Act 1986 is an awkward compendium of amendments to these two Acts, which the British government was required to pass to comply with European Community (EC) legislation. The Race Relations Act 1976 is the sole act covering discrimination on the basis of race, and includes prohibitions regarding discriminatory pay differentials.

The race and sex laws cover a wide range of issues. Since the overwhelming focus of legal activity has been in the employment area, this is considered at some length in this chapter, before we turn to the impact of the laws on housing, education and state activities. The chapter concludes with a description of the significant influence of European law on British equality legislation.

Employment

Few would dispute that women and black people continue to face both widespread discrimination and disadvantage in employment. The most extensive research into the operation of racial discrimination was carried out by the Policy Studies Institute in 1984–5.[1] Controlled testing revealed that over a third of employers who advertised vacancies discriminated against Afro-Caribbean and Asian job applicants. This study measured direct discrimination at the initial stage of hiring only. Adding to this the estimated numbers of indirect discrimination cases indicates that, even on a conservative estimate, there are thousands of acts of race discrimination in job recruitment alone every year.

The most glaring evidence of continuing racial discrimination is the enormous differentials in rates of unemployment: the ethnic minority unemployment rate is 60 per cent above that for whites.[2] Whilst women do not suffer disproportionate rates of unemployment, the huge discrepancy in the rates of pay between the genders bears witness to women's continuing subordination in the labour market: women have continued to earn 70 pence for every £1 paid to men since the late 1970s.[3]

The two central reasons for the failure of sex and race legislation to counter discrimination more effectively in employment are the restricted definition of discrimination and inadequate enforcement mechanisms.

Indirect discrimination

Chapter 2 emphasised the centrality of indirect discrimination to the perpetuation of racial disadvantage, and the importance of this legal concept for challenging it. The Commission for Racial Equality (CRE), in its *Second Review of the Race Relations Act*, shares this assessment:

> Formal investigations have shown that the practices which most affect ethnic minorities' job prospects when the workforce is largely white are those such as recruiting wholly by word of mouth, giving preference to children of existing employees for apprenticeships or only trawling vacancies internally. None of these practices are essential for business efficiency, although there are obviously arguments in their favour; but there is an obvious tendency towards inefficiency by narrowly restricting when there are many others in the job market.[4]

The concept of indirect discrimination, by seeking to go beyond individual complaints, attempts to address the pervasive and systemic nature of discrimination. In Britain, however, the impact of this provision is blunted by the absence of group procedures and by inadequate remedies. No damages are available, unless the discrimination can be shown to be deliberate.[5] Although the complainant is required to show that he or she is a member of a group adversely affected by a particular rule, s/he must argue that position as an individual. If the action is successful then the rule must be changed and others will benefit.[6]

Initially it appeared that the concept would succeed in dismantling some of the structural barriers faced by women and ethnic minorities. An important early victory involved applicants for direct entry to the Executive Grade of the Civil Service. All applicants were required to be under the age of 28. Ms Price complained, and won her case, on the basis that fewer women than men were able to comply with this requirement, because many women brought up children and were out of the labour market during their twenties.[7]

This was followed by a positive ruling in the key area of part-time employment. A civil servant asked to be allowed to return to work on a part-time basis after pregnancy. This was refused on the basis that there were no part-time posts in her grade. The Employment Appeal Tribunal (EAT) ruled that she had been the victim of indirect discrimination.[8] The judge was careful to point out that all such cases would turn on their particular facts, and that the ruling imposed no blanket requirement on all employers to provide part-time employment in this situation. Such reluctance to set broad-reaching standards has been typical of the judiciary's timid approach to this area. This attitude is not surprising in the light of the legal history described in Chapter 5, and has led to widely varying decisions according to the disposition of the presiding judges.

One potentially radical decision ruled that selecting part-timers for redundancy before full-time workers constituted indirect discrimination because of the preponderance of women who worked part-time.[9] However, a completely contradictory decision was subsequently upheld by a different EAT.[10] This lack of consistency is unsatisfactory both for the individuals involved and because it limits the ability of case law to promote clear guidance for promoting equal opportunities.

The decisions of the Court of Appeal have scarcely been more helpful in setting a positive framework to guide tribunals' interpretations of indirect discrimination:

> The judgements of the Court of Appeal were consistently negative. As a result of the Court's intervention, the provision which gave an employer the chance to justify the discriminatory practice became a gaping hole through which almost any complaint of indirect discrimination could be lost.[11]

The definition of 'justifiable' set down by the Court of Appeal exemplifies the unthinking racial bias referred to by Fitzpatrick:[12] 'If a person produces reasons for doing something which would be acceptable to right-thinking people as sound, tolerable reasons for so doing then he has justified his conduct.'[13] The unspoken assumption is that these right-thinking people are white (and naturally also male). 'Justifiable' was subsequently and no more helpfully defined by the House of Lords as 'capable of being justified'.[14]

Happily, European law has forced a more vigorous approach on to the reluctant British judiciary (see pp. 126–8 below for a broader discussion of the powers of the EC to intervene in this area). The

European Court of Justice (ECJ) required that where practices produce adverse effects on one sex, the responsible organisation must prove that it had 'objectively justified reasons' for these practices.[15] A British judgement subsequently elaborated: 'justifiable requires an objective balance between the discriminatory effect of the condition and the reasonable needs of the person who applies the condition.'[16] Despite this improvement, this area of law is likely to continue to be problematic, as discussed in Chapter 2, because of the dominance of the profit motive over alternative considerations.

The first House of Lords case on employment discrimination produced a further damaging restriction on the scope of indirect discrimination by ruling that only requirements or conditions which were an 'absolute bar' to appointment, not merely one factor amongst others, could constitute indirect discrimination.[17] Thus, if a criterion puts ethnic minority applicants (or women) at a significant disadvantage but may be overcome by an individual with exceptional compensatory qualities, such a criterion will be lawful. Both the CRE and the Equal Opportunities Commission (EOC) have proposed reforming the concept of indirect discrimination so that it would include any practice with a significantly adverse impact on members of one sex or one racial group, which could not be shown to be necessary.[18]

These restrictions have effectively checked the concept's radical potential, and it has become little used in the employment area. Only 2 per cent of cases reported to the CRE between 1986 and 1988 related to indirect discrimination, whereas in 1984 they represented 13 per cent of complaints.[19] Formal investigations in the employment area have also tended to focus on direct discrimination. The concept of indirect discrimination has, however, proved crucial in challenging actions in the areas of education, housing and public provision of services, particularly by local authorities, and the EOC has also used it to scrutinise legislative provisions before the European Court (see pp. 126–8 below).

Enforcement
The race relations laws of the 1960s had used an administrative method of enforcement, with all complaints being handled by the Race Relations Board. In contrast, the Equal Pay Act 1970 relied solely on individual complaints, with victims having direct access to the courts. The evident weaknesses in both models prompted the framers of the Sex Discrimination Act (SDA) and Race Relations Act (RRA) to combine both methods of enforcement. Individuals had the right to take legal proceedings on their own behalf, but in addition two Commissions were established (the Equal Opportunities Commission and the Commission for Racial Equality) with broad-reaching powers of investigation and enforcement. Although appointed by the Secretary of State and funded

by the state, these Commissions were intended to act autonomously of the government of the day, accountable ultimately to Parliament.

The Commissions were intended to take a strategic approach to persuading organisations to adopt positive policies. Promotional work was to be backed by their new powers to carry out formal investigations, and they were also required to support individual complaints both for their own sake and as a campaigning resource to change policies and behaviour.

The Commissions can serve notices requiring information which can be made the subject of a binding court order. As the outcome of a formal investigation, the Commissions can issue a non-discrimination notice, requiring a person not to commit specified acts of discrimination, and giving details of the change of policy or practice required by the Commission to avoid future discrimination. Appeal against a non-discrimination notice is available to the High Court. Where the Commission has reasonable cause to believe a notice will not be complied with, it can apply to the court for an order. However, such orders do not have the effect of an injunction, with the only sanction for non-compliance being a small fine. Injunctions are only available if a non-discrimination notice has been issued, and it appears that unless restrained the subject of that order is likely to commit further discriminatory acts in future.

Individual employment cases under the Acts are brought before industrial tribunals, with a limited rights of appeal to EATs. Industrial tribunals have a legally qualified chair, and one member each from the organisations of employers and employees. Where a complaint is upheld, the tribunal can award damages, make a declaration of the rights of parties or make a recommendation that the employer take action to remove or reduce the effect of discrimination on the individual who has complained. However, the scope for changing the practices of an organisation though individual tribunal cases is strictly limited. Even with regard to the individual applicant, the tribunal has no power to 'recommend' that he or she be given priority in respect of future similar jobs, nor that an employer should increase a person's wages.[20]

The methods available to tribunals in order to enforce their decisions are inadequate. Injunctions and contempt powers are not generally available to tribunals, and recommendations are not enforceable; if an employer fails to comply the tribunal can merely increase the damages award.

In non-employment cases, proceedings must be brought in the county court, claiming compensation in the same way as if for a 'tort' (civil wrong). The court can impose injunctions and award damages.

Litigation by individuals

Most of those who experience discrimination do nothing about it. Since we know that discrimination is occurring on a wide scale, the numbers of people using the individual complaints procedures can be taken as an indication of the success of the law in inviting individuals to seek legal redress. The numbers of individual complaints under the RRA represent a substantial improvement on the position under the Race Relations Act 1968. However, for both sex and race commentators are unanimous that the system is inadequate – particularly for unrepresented complainants:

> The number of cases, and the number of successful cases has risen sharply in recent years; this in spite of the fact that the procedure is troublesome, the applicant has a poor prospect of obtaining a small reward, and the present capacity to provide competent representation to applicants is too small to meet the demand.[21]

Discrimination claims have a lower success rate than those for unfair dismissal, and the chances of winning a race discrimination claim are about half that of winning a sex discrimination claim. In 1990–1 out of 1,078 completed sex discrimination cases: 86 were upheld, 206 were dismissed, 384 were settled and 370 were withdrawn. The comparable figures for the RRA were: 47 upheld, 323 dismissed, 185 settled and 371 withdrawn, out of a total of 926 cases.

Few of those who did complain had recourse to a lawyer, although British studies confirm the importance of representation.[22] American research clearly indicates that complainants in class actions are substantially more likely to win,[23] as are those supported by the federal government[24] or interest groups. Commentators agree on the urgent need to extend legal aid to complainants in industrial tribunals:

> Every research study ... reaches the same conclusion: without an adequate system of support and representation, it is virtually impossible for an employee to enter this procedural minefield and emerge triumphant at the other end with a decision in his or her favour.[25]

Providing legal aid for adequate legal representation would also enable the Commissions to choose to represent only those cases which contribute to their role as a strategic enforcement agency.

Quality of decisions

Even with adequate legal representation for applicants, the quality of decisions by the tribunals would remain poor. Leonard's study of all tribunal decisions concerning equal pay and sex discrimination, in three successive years from 1982, found widely varying decisions and a number of cases where the law appeared to have been misinterpreted.[26]

Both Commissions, as well as critics of the Acts, stress the need for specialist tribunals with adequate training.

Of even greater significance, tribunals must become more representative of those who bring complaints before them. At present, for example, only 2.7 per cent of tribunal members are from ethnic minorities,[27] and we saw in Chapter 5 that the situation is even more serious with regard to judges. Bindman, commentating on the prejudices of the judiciary, emphasises the need to revise the way that both judges and tribunal members are selected and trained.[28] Fitzpatrick goes further: 'It is not a matter of a remediable bias or some such. It is a matter of a whole sensibility. Adjudicators cannot be responsive to interests they cannot comprehend.'[29] A Court of Appeal judgement vividly illustrates this lack of empathy. The judge ruled: 'It is impossible to say that the use of the phrase "wog" by one manager to another, even though overheard by the appellant, could properly be described as a "detriment".'[30] It is difficult to imagine a comment more calculated to destroy the relationship of trust between employee and manager.

Damages

A further consequence of the small proportion of those discriminated against who take legal action is that employers are less likely to be influenced by the possibility of a successful complaint. Even where an applicant is successful, the deterrent effect is not likely to be great because the damages awarded are too low. Raising the level of damages awarded would not only raise the stakes involved for firms caught discriminating, but would also increase the incentive to individuals to use the law.

An article discussing employment discrimination against HIV positive people made this point with regard to the unfair dismissal legislation (the only British legislation offering any sort of legal protection):

> The fact is that it is very cheap to pay someone off under the present rules. The maximum amount an employee can be awarded ... for unfair dismissal is £11,000 ... Rather than bring in specific discrimination legislation ... increasing the maximum compensations of industrial tribunals would do far more to prevent employers behaving unfairly.[31]

Damages are available to compensate for pecuniary loss, and for injury to feelings. Damages cannot be awarded where the indirect discrimination is unintentional.[32] Compensatory damages may include an element of 'aggravated damages', where the defendant has acted in a high-handed, malicious or insulting manner.[33] Exemplary damages (the equivalent of punitive damages in America) are also available, but only in rare cases.[34]

Until recently damages have been very low. For example in 1985 a young man who lost his Youth Training Scheme (YTS) placement as a result of discrimination and was said to be 'shattered' received only £30 damages.[35] Gregory's appraisal is difficult to contradict: 'Given the amount of time and trouble involved, it is surprising that so many applicants persist.'[36] Between 1990 and 1993 there was an increase of one-third in the level of awards.[37] But the average award remains low at £1,355, well below the awards made to victims of religious discrimination in Northern Ireland.[38]

One factor contributing to the low levels of awards has been the statutory ceiling on compensation (£11,000). The ECJ has recently ruled that this statutory restraint on damages is in breach of the EC Equal Treatment Directive.[39] Although this ruling relates only to sex discrimination, the Home Secretary announced in late 1993 that the limit will be removed for both sex and race awards.[40] For such a change to have a full impact it would have to go hand in hand with the improved quality of decision-making outlined above. At present, whilst tribunals are limited in the amount of compensation they award, most awards are nowhere near this limit.

Individual law suits have played a significant role in promoting 'group justice' in the United States. Tribunals should be seen not just as a way of resolving individual grievances but also as a way of encouraging change in organisations. The CRE has stressed the importance of recognising the group nature of discrimination.[41] It considers that the British system of adjudication entirely fails to do this, and proposes a series of changes. First, groups of individuals who share a common legal interest should be entitled to take joint legal action. In addition, tribunals should be given powers to award compensation to anyone who it finds has suffered unlawful discrimination and who joins the proceedings. It should also be able to order positive action to deal with the discriminatory situation. At present, even where an individual applicant is successful, the tribunal has no power to order the discriminating organisation to change its ways, never mind prescribe positive action programmes as occurs in America.

Positive action
Chapter 2 discussed the importance of positive action measures to achieve practical results. Meehan's comparative study of British and American equality laws found consensus amongst officials in the US and pressure groups in Britain that 'the faster rate of American desegregation owes a good deal to enforceable affirmative action policies.'[42] In Britain, positive action has been much less widely used. Courts have no power to order affirmative action remedies against discrimination. In addition, the lower financial costs involved in losing a discrimina-

tion case do not provide the incentive for organisations to adopt positive action.

The SDA and RRA only permit positive action in very restricted circumstances. Training bodies and employers are allowed to provide training for members of one particular racial group or sex if there is evidence that those groups are underrepresented in the occupations for which the training is intended,[43] and a number of cases have been successfully brought against organisations seeking to practise positive 'discrimination' in other circumstances – for example, only considering ethnic minority candidates for apprenticeships.

Some local authorities during the 1980s established contract compliance programmes, attempting to use their purchasing power to influence the companies with which they did business. A number sought to impose equal opportunities requirements on contractors. There was some evidence of initial success,[44] but before these had had a chance to achieve any significant progress, the Local Government Act 1988 was introduced. This severely restricts such policies as regards race, and prohibits them totally with regard to sex.[45]

Impact on employers

A number of detailed case studies of individual employers in the United States, looking at the impact of enforcement action, conclude that litigation is the necessary, though not sufficient, tool for promoting change. Litigation and civil rights activism are needed as a lever to persuade employers that it is in their interest not to discriminate.

A study of five employers in the shipbuilding industry highlighted the importance of the threat of losing government contract work.[46] Another study of the successful promotion of employment of black and women workers emphasised the key role an enforcement agency (in this case the EEOC) could play – provided that its threats had sufficient weight.[47] Further research establishes that stricter enforcement mechanisms have considerably more impact than mere persuasion, exemplified by the fact that until the EEOC was given enforcement powers in 1972 it had little success in securing voluntary compliance, in marked contrast to its later success.[48]

British research into the sex discrimination legislation concludes:

There is not much evidence to indicate that an isolated tribunal decision will by itself have enormous repercussions. However, if the organisation or a section of it is favourably disposed to promoting equality of opportunity within the organisation, and if the case is followed up either by a trade union, by the applicant or by the EOC the tribunal decision can be a building block or starting point for further activity.[49]

The research studied 40 organisations who had lost sex discrimination or equal pay cases. In 70 per cent of cases no change in attitudes was detected. *Racial Justice at Work* looks at ten employers who experienced the enforcement procedures of the Race Relations Act to assess whether these mechanisms succeeded in promoting equal opportunities and discouraging discrimination.[50] It concludes that 'changes were generated by contact with enforcement procedures'.[51] This process focused attention beyond the individual complaint. The authors contrast individual cases with strategic investigations: 'Tribunals tend on their own to produce less comprehensive approaches to change than investigations do. Tribunals promote urgent action whereas investigations promote more considered action.'[52]

Strategic investigations

The Commissions also have the power to initiate legal proceedings on their own behalf in cases of persistent or continuing discrimination, but only in the area of employment.

Both Commissions are authorised to conduct formal investigations for any purpose connected with its statutory duties; an individual complaint is not required to trigger an investigation. Non-discrimination notices can be issued where there is evidence of unlawful discrimination. But such notices can only restrain organisations from future unlawful acts, not prescribe positive action policies. Once again this is a crucial area of weakness in the operation of the Acts. The scope of this enforcement mechanism has also been severely restricted by judicial interpretation. The House of Lords has ruled that the CRE is not entitled to conduct investigations into the activity of specific organisations unless it has reason to believe that unlawful discrimination might be occurring.[53]

Up to this House of Lords case the CRE had been very active (indeed a Commons Committee had reprimanded it for overstretching its resources and failing to select strategic targets). Partly as a result of the legal restrictions imposed on it, the CRE cut back drastically on the number of its employment investigations. Strategic enforcement through formal investigations was effectively curtailed by the difficulties which previous investigations had encountered in the courts. It made some use of general investigations, but these are apt to become broad and diffuse.

The EOC had in any event carried out fewer investigations. Indeed, Gregory comments that: 'The timidity and indecision of the Commission in Manchester contrasts sharply with the almost frenzied activities of the Commission for Racial Equality in London.'[54] Undoubtedly, it was also deterred by these adverse judicial decisions. Perhaps owing to its lower level of resources, the EOC has concentrated on promotional activity rather than adversarial investigations. However, as *Racial Justice at Work* points out, the efficacy of such activity would also be affected by the blunting of formal enforcement powers:

> The power to initiate formal investigations provides an incentive for bargaining. There is, however, a vital distinction between bargaining from a position of strength (where launching a formal investigation into a specified organisation and issuing a non-discrimination notice is a real threat) and bargaining from a position of weakness.[55]

The authors of this in-depth analysis of the operation of the RRA argue that as the credible negotiating stance built up by the first generation of investigations wore off, the CRE was increasingly negotiating from a position of weakness. Whilst they accept that in some cases publicity itself is a sanction, they stress that for the strategic investigative powers of the Commission to function effectively its bargaining position must be improved by increasing the Commission's statutory powers. Specifically, they point to the enforcement structure of the Fair Employment Commission, which acts against religious discrimination in Northern Ireland. This involves compulsory monitoring requirements for employers, increased remedial powers, the ability to require affirmative action remedies, the imposition of goals and timetables and increased sanctions for non-compliance, including the possible loss of government contracts and grants.

Monitoring
The CRE, in its *Second Review of the Race Relations Act*, points to the provisions in Northern Ireland as an indication of the mechanisms which are required in the rest of the United Kingdom. The organisation particularly stresses the need for ethnic monitoring, quoting the Standing Advisory Committee on Human Rights:

> Anti-discrimination agencies in every jurisdiction of which the Committee is aware now regard monitoring, both of the composition of the workforce as a whole and of the results of recruitment and promotion, to be an essential tool in controlling discrimination and promoting equality of opportunity.[56]

The CRE argues that monitoring is the only mechanism that will detect the covert and often unintentional discrimination which plays such a powerful part in keeping black people (and all those discriminated against) subordinate. It describes the principal purpose of monitoring as making an employer aware of the situation within his or her workforce, to enable him or her to take action. 'The Race Relations Act 1976 relies entirely on voluntary action to achieve change, provided only that employers avoid actual racial discrimination.'[57] Compulsory monitoring would help move beyond this narrow, negative concept to a more effective practice of equal opportunities, with the positive goal of 'fair' participation.

Fair Employment (Northern Ireland) Act 1989

It is interesting to look at this recent Act, as it contains many of the provisions which reformers of the SDA and RRA are seeking.[58] Complaints are heard by a specialised tribunal, and the limit for compensation for individuals is £30,000. Public sector employers and many private sector employers are required to register with the Fair Employment Commission and to review their practices periodically. They are required to monitor the religious composition of their workforces, with detailed forms including breakdowns of the religious composition of different occupations and applicants. Where imbalances are evident, employers are required to engage in affirmative action; this is enforceable by the Commission, which can set goals and timetables. The Commission has broader powers than those of the CRE or EOC. It can review patterns of employment without needing to have specific suspicion of discrimination, and can accept binding and enforceable agreements from employers. Finally, government contracts and funding can be withdrawn from firms which fail to cooperate in promoting equal opportunities.

Appointment to the Commissions

Aside from the issue of the powers of the Commissions, questions have been raised about their composition and their capacity to act as independent pressure groups capable of producing tangible benefits. The issue has been raised particularly with respect to the EOC, perceived as being a less vigorous champion of the cause of equality.

Blumenrosen, a former senior staff member of the American EEOC, argues that administrators must go beyond 'bland neutrality', by involving the protected class, if the resistance of regulated groups is to be overcome.[59] In contrast, EOC appointments have been handed out as political favours, rewarding prominent people for contributions to political parties and areas of public life. More problematic still is the policy of including representatives of vested interests. The Trades Union Congress (TUC) and Confederation of British Industry (CBI) have three nominations each on to the EOC (two each on to the CRE). Meehan argues, unsurprisingly, that they use their positions to preserve the status quo.[60] One TUC appointment lost her union job and was removed from the Commission for refusing to follow the union line.[61] Gregory argues that it is precisely these nominees who tend to dominate the Commission, as the others are part-time and not linked to particular constituencies:

Most commissioners have been minor figures with dubious credentials for the job. It has been a huge mistake, and it was clearly a deliberate decision, not to include in the membership of the Commission some credible leaders of the women's movement who had some knowledge and understanding of the issues ... The effect ... has been the worse because the Commissioners ... have not been held accountable to anyone, formally or informally. This enabled the CBI and TUC to exercise disproportionate influence which has generally been cautious, defensive and at times destructive.[62]

Both authors argue that appointments have steered clear of women committed to female equality. One ex-Commissioner, quoted by Gregory, thought that this practice might constitute indirect sex discrimination,[63] and in fact two cases have been brought by women against the EOC for alleged employment discrimination, one by a Commissioner and the other by a senior member of staff.

A recent British attempt to pass anti-discrimination legislation for disabled people, the Civil Rights (Disabled Persons) Bill 1993, sought to address this issue by requiring that at least three-quarters of the Commissioners of a future Disability Commission should themselves be disabled. There was also a recognition amongst the proponents of the legislation that such people should be representative of, and to the maximum extent possible accountable to, the disability movement. It may be easier to achieve this in the disability area since, if the legislation is modelled on the American Act, it will specifically protect disabled people from discrimination. In contrast, the SDA and the RRA are both couched in neutral terms, requiring equal treatment for all, and the Commissions are correspondingly unable to cast themselves purely as the champions of particular sections of society.

Non-employment provisions

The Acts prohibit discrimination in education, housing and the provision of 'goods, facilities and services'.[64] This last term is defined by a non-exhaustive list: hotels, banking, insurance, credit facilities and 'other financial services' cinemas, theatres, restaurants, pubs and other places offering public entertainment or refreshment, facilities for transport and travel, and services provided by any trade or profession, or by any local or public authority. It is unlawful for such organisations to discriminate by refusing services, or by providing them on less favourable conditions than those offered to people of the opposite sex or another racial group. Both Acts originally exempted 'private' transactions, such as those offered by private clubs. Interestingly, the Race Relations Act was amended so that private clubs now fall within its ambit if they have 25 or more members, but despite attempts by the EOC the ambit of the SDA has not been similarly extended.

The primary emphasis of both Commissions has been in the employment area:

> Employment was the first priority of the Commission's investiga-
> tion strategy because of its importance to the black community and
> the widespread extent of discrimination substantiated by PEP research,
> and also because it was regarded as particularly open to investiga-
> tion: indeed the whole argument for the need for investigative
> powers was originally formulated in the context of employment.[65]

Although employment is by far the largest category of complaints brought by individuals to the Commissions, large numbers of individuals have complained about discrimination outside employment. In 1992, for example, the EOC received 1,903 complaints about education and training, 1,001 about goods, facilities and services and 2,233 about 'family policy', which covers issues such as parental rights, childcare and alternative working arrangements. Other significant categories of complaints included retirement (218) and pension provisions (368).[66]

It is misleading to judge the significance of issues in perpetuating sex and race discrimination solely from the volume of complaints. To a great extent the degree to which people seek legal recourse will depend on their evaluation, first, of their own interest in challenging a particular act of discrimination and, second, of the degree to which it is possible legally to challenge that act. A discriminatory service may have a significant impact in perpetuating sexism or racism, but for indi-viduals the stakes may not be high enough to take action. For example, if it is open to individuals to resolve a problem by seeking a service from an alternative source they are less likely to challenge the original source legally.

The role of indirect discrimination, which by its nature tends to be opaque to individual challenge, is strong in service provision. For individuals this is experienced as a strong feeling that discrimination is happening, while being unable to pinpoint precisely where in the system, or how it happens. For example, a formal investigation into the practices of one local education authority (LEA) revealed that Afro-Caribbean pupils were four times more likely than white pupils to be suspended from schools for similar offences.[67] The many significant aspects of the covert sexism and racism of the education system are not, however, amenable to individual challenge.

In addition, the inaccessibility of the legal system for challenging certain forms of discrimination has a significant effect in discourag-ing complaints:

Since the introduction of the Sex Discrimination Act only a handful of the thousands of complaints in the field of education and consumer services has reached the county courts. Complainants can be deterred from pursuing cases by the formality, procedural complications and expense involved.[68]

These factors make the role of strategic actors like the Commissions vital in these areas. The CRE has been particularly active in scrutinising the services provision of local authorities – housing, education and social services – and has also worked in the areas of the media, adoption, the criminal justice system and the health service.

Of the 46 investigations begun by the CRE between 1977 and 1981, 24 involved employment, 2 involved education, 11 were in housing, eight in the provision of goods, facilities and services and 1 in immigration.

Since 1983 the number of formal investigations has fallen and the proportion has altered: 7 were started by the employment section, 5 in education, 1 in the provision of goods and services and 7 in housing. McCrudden et al suggest that this was, in part, the result of the far greater number of individual complainants in employment compared to housing: 'Much of the enforcement activity in the employment sphere therefore takes place in tribunals ... Much of this enforcement activity through industrial tribunals in the field of employment was replaced by investigations of organisations in the field of housing.'[69]

The CRE has been much more active outside the employment area than the EOC has. To a great extent this must be attributable to its substantially greater resources – the CRE received a grant of £11,727,606 in 1989/90, compared to £3,955,763 for the EOC. The EOC lack of action outside of employment, and to a lesser extent education, is also attributable to discrepancies in the legal reach of the two anti-discrimination acts. Whilst the SDA contains an express prohibition on discrimination in the services of any local or public authority (s. 29), the EOC does not regard this as adequate to deal with the issues that arise. It proposes imposing a duty on local authorities similar to that already contained within the RRA, requiring local authorities to have 'due regard' to the need to eliminate racial discrimination and 'to promote equality of opportunity, and good relations, between persons of different racial groups'.[70]

Even if no actual discrimination occurs, the way in which local authorities and other public bodies provide their services can have a great influence on the opportunities in practice available to women: for example, the services provided for those having the responsibility to care either for young children or for elderly and disabled relatives (predominantly women) can have a significant effect on their ability to enter employment. Women are also more dependent than men on public transport, and the availability ... of adequate transport can equally strongly influence the extent to which they can undertake employment or other activities outside the home.[71]

In looking at the activities of the Commissions it is as well to bear in mind that these will also reflect the different pattern of discrimination which arises when considering issues of race and gender. Were a Disability Commission to be set up, with the same sort of powers as those of the CRE and EOC, it would inevitably highlight different areas, most obviously the issue of physical access to public buildings and transport systems. However, an examination of the enforcement of anti-discrimination provisions in the areas of housing and education can give an insight into a future Disability Commission's role in these areas.

Housing

The CRE has been active in the housing area, particularly with regard to local authorities,[72] making important use of the concept of indirect discrimination. Its investigations have certainly revealed significant amounts of direct discrimination by housing officials, but have also focused on the institutional processes which have led larger proportions of black people to be excluded entirely from access to local authority housing, or confined them to the worse estates. One factor is the shortage of larger properties, which has a disproportionate effect because on average black families are larger in size.[73] The prevalence of racial harassment in certain all-white estates has also had a powerful effect, leading some local authorities to react by excluding black families from those estates and confining them to 'ghetto' estates, of invariably inferior standards.[74]

Henderson and Karn, in their study of Birmingham's council housing policy, have found additional policies which disadvantage Afro-Caribbean and Asian families: a requirement that applicants be resident in the city for at least five years, and the disqualification of single people, militates against newcomers; the disqualification of applications by owner–occupiers discriminates against black people, who are more likely than white people to be in low-income owner–occupation; the rejection of applications by joint families fails to take into account the different household structure in the Asian community; whilst restrictions on applications by unmarried couples show a similar failure towards the Afro-Caribbean community.[75]

The concentration of research on public sector housing does not indicate that the private sector is free from discriminatory attitudes. The CRE discovered institutionalised racism in the practices of estate agents in Oldham,[76] and of lenders in Rochdale.[77]

Ginsburg discusses how, with the law as an underpinning and incentive, effective anti-racist policies can be developed.[78] The CRE established guidelines for local authority policies in its report of its investigation into Hackney's policies.[79]

Education

The education provisions of the sex and race acts make unlawful specified types of discrimination by certain bodies in charge of educational establishments. Discrimination is defined as refusing to admit applicants, or admitting them on discriminatory terms. It also includes denying pupils access to 'benefits, facilities or services' or offering them access on discriminatory terms; or by excluding pupils or 'subjecting him/her to any other detriment'.[80] In addition, wider duties are imposed on LEAs not to discriminate in carrying out their functions and to ensure that facilities for education and any ancillary benefits and services are provided without discrimination.[81] These latter provisions are concerned with planning educational provision in such a way as to ensure freedom from discrimination.

Whilst the RRA equates segregation with less favourable treatment,[82] the SDA allows separate facilities for boys and girls in a coeducational school, provided that the facilities for each sex offer equal opportunities. Another interesting difference is that the RRA specifically permits additional services to be offered to persons of a particular racial group in order to meet the 'special needs' of persons of that group in relation to education, training or welfare.[83] Typically special language facilities have been provided under this provision (as have 'special housing needs', or special needs for counselling when starting businesses in other policy areas).

As we will see in Chapter 7, these issues of segregation and provision for meeting 'special needs', and in particular the question of whether meeting 'special needs' justifies segregation, are of crucial importance in the education of disabled children.

As presently constituted, the education provisions restrict the ability of individuals to bring court proceedings, or of the Commissions to issue non-discrimination notices in crucial areas, requiring them to go through the Secretary of State. The CRE has requested that these restrictions be lifted.[84]

Education is recognised by the EOC as a crucial area in which sex discrimination is perpetuated. It has prioritised this for activities, as has the CRE. The EOC conducted one of its rare formal investigations into the publicly funded vocational training system, and both Commissions have brought cases scrutinising the role of LEAs in ensuring equality of provision, despite the advent of educational reforms. In October 1992 the Court of Appeal ruled that in providing sufficient places to ensure suitably qualified boys and girls have equal opportunities, Birmingham City Council was obliged to take account of the availability of places provided by grant-maintained schools in its area. Once again, this issue is likely to be of great significance for the future education of disabled children.

State discrimination

In America the Equal Protection clause of the constitution provides legal protection against race and, to a lesser extent, sex discrimination by the state, and thus provides a principled underpinning for the civil rights legislation which restricts the actions of private individuals and organisations. In Britain, in contrast, not only is there no constitution upon which to base equality principles, but the scope of the legislation is severely restricted with regard to the actions of the state. In particular, those areas which have an especially harsh impact in terms of perpetuating disadvantage, such as social security and immigration, are specifically excluded.

The CRE is very critical of these exemptions:

> ... it sends out the message that the elimination of racial discrimination is not perceived by the Government to be of fundamental importance since there are other concerns to which it must give way ... It is inconsistent with the principles underlying the Act that legislators and ministers should have a free hand to establish systems where racial discrimination can flourish immune from its enforcement provisions.[85]

The SDA gives exemption to all Acts in force at the time of its passage, and for statutory instruments made under those Acts, even if they are made after the SDA was passed.[86] The exemption in the RRA is even broader: all legislation before and after it is exempt, together with circulars guidance and ministerial pronouncements with regard to immigration laws.[87]

The extent to which state actions can be challenged as discriminatory has been restricted still further by judicial interpretation of the Acts. A 1983 House of Lords case, involving a challenge to immigration officials, established that the provisions of the RRA banning discrimination in the provision of goods and services applied only to 'market place activities', and thus many key forms of state provision were placed out of reach by the legislation.[88] The CRE comments that: 'This lack of remedy occurs precisely where the individual is most vulnerable.'[89]

We have already seen that the Race Relations Act imposes certain duties on local authorities, and that this has been useful in facilitating action where the local political will exists. The wording is too vague, however, to enable legal action to be taken to force authorities to act if they would not otherwise have done so. The CRE has therefore asked for this section to be strengthened by placing a positive duty on local authorities to combat discrimination, and by requiring annual programmes.[90] It would also like the duty extended to other local statutory bodies, such as health authorities.

The area of state actions is likely to be particularly important for legislation seeking to combat disability discrimination, given both the importance of state activity for disabled people and the history of state discrimination in the guise of paternalism, described in Chapter 1.

Europe

The constraints imposed on state actions by the SDA and RRA were thus very weak. However, Britain's membership of the European Community has introduced a new external authority, capable of overriding the previously unchallengeable decisions of Parliament. British courts are now obliged to interpret laws in accordance with the broader principles established by European Community law, and their decisions can be appealed to the European Court of Justice. The actions of the EC have played a significant role both in imposing additional restraints on state discrimination and in extending the principles of equality. (Indeed, Britain's forthcoming entry into the EEC was itself an important factor in the passage of the Sex Discrimination Act.)

The chief impact of EC law has been on sex discrimination, because a specific clause of one of the founding treaties addresses this issue directly. Other forms of discrimination are not mentioned in the founding treaties. However, to an extent race discrimination law has been indirectly affected too, by interpretations of key terms in the context of gender discrimination.

Article 119 of the Treaty of Rome requires member states to secure equal treatment between the sexes. It has been given specific implementation in a series of Directives covering equal pay, social security, equal treatment and pregnancy.[91] EC Directives require member states to pass national legislation to give effect to their objectives, and these Directives have been implemented in Britain by the Social Security Act 1980, the Sex Discrimination Act 1986 and the Trade Union Reform and Employment Rights Act 1993.

Britain has 'adopted a minimalist position, making the smallest number of changes necessary to comply with European law'.[92] Thus, for example, in response to a European Court of Justice ruling that British law failed to comply with the Equal Pay Directive[93] Parliament introduced amending regulations.[94] However, the resulting procedures were so complicated that only 23 successful cases have been completed since the regulations came into force in 1984. The EOC has argued that the simplification of procedures and the introduction of class actions are essential if this law is not to remain a dead letter, and has asked the European Commission to intervene on the basis that the government has failed to implement the EC Directive.[95]

European law has had a positive effect in expanding the meaning of non-discrimination. We have already seen how this has broadened the concept of indirect discrimination in employment law. O'Donovan and Szyszczak criticise the EC for its failure to move beyond the limited conception of equality, described in Chapter 2 as the formal equality model: 'The resort to biological difference is seen as a justification in several of the provisions for exclusion of the concept of equality rather than coming to terms with accommodating a differences approach.'[96] They point in particular to the exclusions of maternity and pregnancy from the Equal Treatment and Social Security Directive, and to the generally 'timid' approach of the ECJ on these issues. However, since they wrote those comments the EC has taken significant steps to expand its conceptions of equality beyond merely comparing women with a similarly situated man. This comparative approach has most obviously stretched credulity in the area of pregnancy, and it is here that the EC has recently moved beyond the 'assimilationist approach'. In the Dekker case,[97] the complainant was rejected for the post of training instructor, despite the fact that she was a suitably qualified candidate, on the sole basis that she was pregnant. The ECJ ruled unequivocally that:

> As employment can only be refused because of pregnancy to women, such a refusal is direct discrimination on grounds of sex ... Such discrimination cannot be justified by the financial detriment in the case of a pregnant woman suffered by her employer during her maternity leave.[98]

Despite this seemingly definitive ruling, the British Court of Appeal in a subsequent case managed to continue to permit decisions based solely on the basis of pregnancy, at least in the private sector where provisions of the Equal Treatment Directive do not directly apply.[99] This ruling has since been superseded by further EC intervention. A Pregnancy Directive was issued in October 1992 requiring member states to make provision for 14 weeks paid maternity leave and protection from dismissal by reason of pregnancy from the inception of employment. The British government chose to implement the minimum provisions required under this Directive in the Trade Union Reform and Employment Rights Act 1993. The EOC criticised this grudging implementation as encouraging discrimination, by requiring employers to contribute to maternity pay. The Institute of Directors appeared to concur, warning that employers would be cautious about employing young women if they were forced to bear additional costs.

The EC has been more tentative when applying the concept of indirect discrimination, since the 'economic factors' defence is much harder to apply in areas where the state is making decisions. Nevertheless, the ECJ has laid down some legislative provision on the basis of indirect discrimination, and has even been prepared to rule in the complex area of social security that member states have breached the Social Security Directive on the grounds of direct sex discrimination: 'the Court has cut through complex arguments of economic costs and the acceptance of discriminatory systems of benefits based on stereotyped notions of married women's role in the family and the labour market.'[100]

In addition, in 1994 the House of Lords ruled that the statutory exclusions of part-time workers in respect of unfair dismissal and redundancy rights constituted indirect discrimination under European Community law, since women predominate in part-time work and are adversely affected by these restrictions.[101] This decision will result in the invaluable extension of legal protection to many vulnerable female workers for the first time.

Conclusion

There is a considerable degree of consensus amongst those researching the processes of discrimination about the need to improve the operation of the SDA and RRA. There is also considerable agreement about the types of changes which are required. Improving individual access to justice by extending legal aid; improving the quality of judicial decisions by increased training and representativeness of tribunal members and judges; and strengthening strategic enforcement efforts by making provision for group actions and group remedies, including the power to order positive action and extending the scope of formal investigations, are all acknowleged to be of crucial importance. Also recognised is the need to strengthen the definition of indirect discrimination and provide higher damages, as a disincentive to discriminators. Greater accountability of the Commissions and extending the reach of anti-discrimination law over a broader range of state activities are likely to be particularly important to disabled people.

7
Restructuring British Disability Laws

The introductory chapter gave a rather caricatured description of the British legislative approach to disability, contrasting its welfarist approach to the rights-based American model. The contrast is somewhat less sharp than that chapter implied, since there are scattered glimpses of a rights-based approach in British legislation since 1970. In this chapter I consider how these diffuse strands might be built upon and developed into comprehensive anti-discrimination legislation.

Civil Rights (Disabled Persons) Bill 1993

There have been eleven attempts to pass anti-discrimination legislation for people with disabilities in Britain, and the background to these is examined in more detail in Chapter 8. The most recent attempt, the Civil Rights (Disabled Persons) Bill 1993, was also the most detailed proposal, and as such an essential starting point for any discussion of the shape which British anti-discrimination legislation might take. The Bill married key concepts from the Americans with Disabilities Act with the enforcement mechanisms of the British sex and race discrimination legislation. The definition of disability was identical to that used in the ADA.

The debt to the ADA was most obvious in the employment section, which was considerably more detailed than sections covering other provisions. The Bill would have banned direct and indirect discrimination, and qualification standards or selection tests which screen out disabled people unless they could be shown to be essential to the job for which they are required. In addition, employers would have been required to provide reasonable accommodation for applicants or employees (unless this would unduly prejudice an employer) to be assessed by reference to the cost of the actions, taking into account the availability of public subsidies, weighed against the resources of the covered entity.

As with the ADA, the Civil Rights Bill would not have applied to small employers; only firms with 20 or more employees would have been covered. There are good grounds for taking a less cautious approach and extending protection against disability discrimination to all employees and applicants, regardless of the size of the employing organisation. Limitations regarding the extent of modifications required already exist by virtue of the provision concerning 'undue predjudice'. It is surely wrong in principle for someone's civil right to be contingent on the size of a company, and no such restriction applies to the sex or race discrimination laws.

The section concerning goods and services was rather more sketchy. Part III[1] provided that no 'qualified disabled person' should be denied participation in, or the benefits of, services or programmes in a broad spectrum of areas: education, recreation, the provision of goods, facilities and services, insurance, transport, housing and accommodation, occupational pension schemes, membership of clubs and associations and civic rights and duties. In determining whether or not someone met the essential eligibility requirements for such services, the provision of reasonable modifications was to be taken into account where required by a person's disability. Reasonable modification would have been required to 'rules, policies or practices', as would the 'removal of architectural, communication or transport barriers', and 'the provision of auxiliary aids and services'. Such actions would not have been required if they entailed 'undue hardship', to be assessed in the same way as undue prejudice, that is by reference to the cost of the actions, taking into account the availability of public subsidies, weighed against the resources of the covered entity.

It would have remained lawful to deny access to services and activities if this were 'impracticable or unsafe', but only if access could not be rendered safe and practicable by reasonable modifications. Whilst, with the provision of appropriate guidelines, it is acceptable that safety should be taken into account, the concept of 'practicability' seems to have been unnecessary and might have led to restrictive interpretations of the scope of the law. Provision was made in the Bill for Codes of Practice to be drawn up, to provide more detailed guidelines on non-discriminatory provision.

One general point which applies to the definition of discrimination provided by the Bill was its failure to include segregation as discriminatory per se. Whilst segregation may be desirable in some instances, it is surely advisable, given the history of enforced exclusion and segregation to which disabled people have been subjected, to regard enforced segregation as discriminatory except in tightly defined circumstances.

Enforcement

As with the sex and race legislation, individuals would have been able to take up their own legal proceedings in tribunals (for employment) and the county court (for other matters). The Commission for Racial Equality (CRE) proposes that all cases of discrimination should be heard in industrial tribunals:[2]

The old Race Relations Board argued powerfully against granting county and sheriff courts jurisdiction in non-employment cases, and it has been proved right. Half the complaints to the old Race Relations Board concerned non-employment matters. Most of the cases which it took to court were non-employment cases ... But under the present Act, the balance has shifted, without any intention on legislators' part that this should happen ... The delays inherent in the court system and the need for legal assistance, all for very low potential award of damages, act as a considerable disincentive to pursuing cases there.[3]

The procedures for tribunals are far more straightforward, and consequently cases tend to be heard more speedily. Alongside this proposal the CRE suggests the establishment of a specialised discrimination tribunal. The one drawback with this is that legal aid is currently available for cases in county courts, but not before tribunals. It would therefore be essential to extend legal aid to tribunal hearings.

The Bill would have established a Disablement Commission, to fulfil the same role as the Equal Opportunities Commission (EOC) and CRE. The crucial enforcement powers of the Commission, however, were to be specified by regulations at a later date. It is important to bear in mind the difficulties which we have seen have been caused by the restrictions on the existing Commissions' powers, and indeed the other improvements outlined in the preceding chapter should also ideally be built into a disability law. It is far more difficult to go back to amend a badly drafted Act than it is to get it right first time.

The intention, given the limited parliamentary time available to any Private Members Bill, was to sketch out the broad legislative approach. The details would then have been filled in during the Committee stage, in subsequent legislative attempts, or by regulations. This chapter considers how this general approach would relate to existing legislation in the areas of access and housing, transport, education and public services, and what further details might usefully be included.

The built environment

The Chronically Sick and Disabled Persons Act 1970 (CSDPA) contained the first explicit consideration in British legislation of the need to open up the built environment to disabled people. Section 4 requires anyone in charge of public buildings to make adequate provision for disabled people with regard to access, toilets and parking facilities. Section 6 extends this requirement to places of accommodation, refreshment or entertainment, whilst Section 8 relates to access and facilities at universities and schools. The Chronically Sick and Disabled Persons

(Amendment) Act 1976 extended these requirements to places of employment.

These provisions contain two fundamental weaknesses. The first is the extremely broad exemptions clause. Provision need only be made if it is 'both reasonable and practicable' to do so, and no further definition of this term is provided. In effect local authorities, who are charged with the responsibility for overseeing this section, are free to interpret it as they please. This first weakness is accentuated by the second: the enforcement of the Act is entirely in the hands of the local authority. Disabled people do not have the power to bring actions against the owners of buildings who fail to comply with the requirement.

On the other hand, the developers of property do have the legal standing to appeal decisions under this Section by the local authority. Topliss and Gould report that, shortly after the Act was passed, an authority's refusal to approve plans for a cinema and supermarket on the basis that Section 4 had not been complied with was overturned on appeal – despite the lack of support for the developer's argument that it was not economical or safe to provide access for disabled people. 'With no other basis on which to determine what was practicable and reasonable in the circumstances, the appeal was allowed, discouraging any further attempts to enforce the access provisions by withholding planning permission.'[4] Topliss and Gould conclude that the waiver clause 'has meant that the needs of disabled persons have continued to be disregarded almost as widely as before'.[5]

Pressure from disability lobbyists resulted in the inclusion of a section on access requirements (Part M) being added to the Building Regulations in 1985. This applies to new public buildings, as well as to substantial extensions to existing buildings. However, many classes of public buildings remain exempt from these requirements, for example British Rail properties, military and agricultural establishments, Crown properties and most educational buildings (which are merely covered by 'guidance' from the Department for Education).

In 1992 the access requirements were extended to incorporate the needs of people with hearing or visual impairments, and applied to all storeys of new buildings. Local authorities have sole responsibility for enforcing Building Regulations.

However, it is not only physical barriers which restrict access by disabled people to the services and places which able-bodied people take for granted. The attitudes of able-bodied people can prove equally restrictive. The Committee on Restrictions against Disabled People (CORAD) Report emphasises the effects of such prejudices:

> ... discrimination is not always inadvertent but is occasionally direct and even hostile in intent. Several people mentioned that they had been refused admission to public houses, for reasons varying from

... that a wheelchair would ruin a new carpet, to the risk of embarrassing other customers ... Correspondents ... wrote of being told 'people like you should stay at home', and of overhearing 'people like them should not be allowed out.'[6]

Nor has the situation improved since that report. Colin Barnes states in his survey of discrimination in Britain, published in 1991:

Discrimination against disabled people within the leisure industry is sometimes quite blatant. It is not uncommon for them to be refused entry to places of entertainment simply because they have an impairment. The usual rationalisation is that their presence prevents non-disabled people from enjoying themselves.[7]

A further common justification is that disabled people pose a safety hazard. Managers of public accommodations frequently refuse to admit unaccompanied blind people or wheelchair users. The CORAD Report quotes the example of a young couple who could not celebrate their wedding anniversary on their own in the theatre because they used wheelchairs; they had to take non-disabled people with them![8]

In theory, current safety and fire regulations represent an improvement. They state that: 'in a society which values the rights and amenities available to all, fire regulations should not be used to place unnecessary restrictions on the ability of disabled persons, particularly those whose mobility is impaired, to use places of entertainment.'[9]

Laudatory as such sentiments are, they cannot be used by disabled people to secure entry into places from which they are excluded. The regulations themselves merely 'recommend' that licensing authorities 'encourage' the licensee to make suitable arrangements. Health and safety are also frequently used as justification for excluding disabled people. Once again, regulations exist, setting out adequate precautions,[10] but are discretionary and therefore largely ignored.

Legal solutions

The Civil Rights Bill would have made such attitudinal prejudice illegal, and would also have required all buildings used for public purposes (public accommodations) to provide access to disabled people unless this could not be achieved without undue hardship. This would have had the advantage of making some impact on improving the accessibility of existing structures. Where access barriers could not be overcome, service providers would have been required to attempt to make alternative provision. For example, if the top floor of a shop could not be rendered accessible shop assistants could bring down goods to disabled customers.

The provision regarding modification to practices would benefit from detailed guidance to businesses, as has been provided in America, although many solutions are simple helpfulness and common sense, for example reading a menu to a blind customer.

The issue of safety could no longer have been used as an excuse to deny access if the Civil Rights Bill had been passed. Although access could have been refused on the basis that it was unsafe, this would not have been permissible if it could have been rendered safe by reasonable modifications to practices, removal of barriers or the provision of auxiliary aids.

An anti-discrimination law should also incorporate the Building Regulations, thus protecting them from future 'deregulation' drives. Incorporating building access requirements into overarching anti-discrimination legislation would also make it clear that such requirements stem from a civil rights imperative. By defining access as a civil right, individuals would be able to sue and claim damages for lack of access to buildings. The content of the regulations should be improved, to include the best principles of accessible design.

The empowerment of individual disabled people (or indeed groups, bringing 'class actions') to take action against offending property owners or occupiers is essential in order to secure effective enforcement of access laws. In addition, damages must be sufficiently high to act as a deterrent, and to secure this guidelines and minimum amounts for damages could be included in regulations.

The capacity of disabled people to bring legal proceedings will naturally be limited by cost, etc., and therefore strategic enforcement by a Disablement Commission is essential. It is also important that local authorities continue to have the power to scrutinise and control building applications to ensure compliance. Indeed, their power could usefully be extended by allowing them to intervene at an early stage of the development. (Building regulations apply when plans are already at a detailed stage, which makes alterations more difficult.) Nevertheless it is crucial to establish the principle that lack of access is an offence against the civil rights of disabled people, and not merely a technical breach of state regulations, with disabled people being mere passive bystanders.

Housing

Part M of the Building Regulations does not apply to housing, and although the CSDPA imposed a duty on local authorities to 'have regard' to the needs of disabled people when planning housing, once again the principle has proved far more significant than the practice.

Significant conceptual and policy advances were, however, made in the 1970s, with the concept of adaptable housing. Adaptable housing, whilst not itself suitable for occupation (as opposed to visits) by wheelchair users, is easily adaptable for such use. The extra cost of such new buildings is negligible compared to the prices of adapting buildings later on.

The 1970s also saw slow but encouraging improvements in the housing policies of local authorities. The CSDPA was followed by a Department of the Environment Circular setting out the specifications of 'mobility housing'.[11] However, these specifications are now 20 years out of date and could usefully be improved. More seriously, the decline in the building of public housing since the early 1980s has effectively halted progress.

As we saw in Chapter 1, there is currently a desperate shortage of accessible homes.[12] Most of the housing stock in the private sector is unsuitable for anyone with mobility impairments. According to Barnes, 'not one major British private housebuilder has adopted the minimum standards for accessible housing, namely mobility standards, and thus the stock of inaccessible housing continues to grow.'[13] Although local authorities have a duty to provide 'Disabled Facilities Grants'[14] to enable dwellings to be adapted to make them suitable for disabled occupants, this help is unavailable in practice to many disabled people, the primary reason being that local authorities require contributions from disabled people which they are frequently unable to pay.[15]

There is clear evidence that large numbers of disabled people live in accommodation which needs adaptation, but they cannot obtain it.[16] Overcrowding, lack of privacy and independence increase discomfort and often create dangers to the health of the disabled person and other occupants. Colin Barnes points out that, even if such grants were readily available, this ad hoc solution fails to address the central issue of discrimination: 'if the only dwellings which are adapted for use by disabled people are their own, then they represent little more than private prisons'.[17]

Added to this massive weight of structural discrimination is overt hostility against some disabled people. This may be reflected in private landlords refusing to rent, for example, to people with Aids, or neighbourhood organisations objecting to the housing of mentally ill or learning disabled persons. A legally sanctioned exercise of prejudice has arisen in the past where covenants attached to property restrict its use. Ian Bynoe has described a case where such a covenant prevented the property being used as 'an asylum for the insane or for the purposes of a hospital for contagious diseases'.[18] An application was made to lift the restriction to enable a children's home to be converted into a home for adults with learning disabilities. The president of the Lands Tribunal refused, and gave the following reason:

The very act of imposing such a covenant discloses the universal abhorrence felt by ordinary folk for the 'mental case' and while that revulsion may derive from ignorance and be justly stigmatised as prejudice it is no less poignant for being unjustified.[19]

Bynoe commented that 'there is still no rule or principle preventing a property owner from refusing the sale or occupation of land' by people with disabilities, and points out that if the judges had seen fit they could have revoked the covenants on the basis that enforcing such prejudice would be contrary to public policy.[20]

A 1993 case, however, produced a different verdict. Neighbours were objecting to a house being used to provide supported housing for discharged psychiatric patients. The Lands Tribunal judge ruled that preventing the conversion was 'contrary to public interest'.[21]

A further, fundamental barrier to housing in the private sector is the low incomes of most disabled people. These make the private rented or owner-occupied sectors difficult to afford.

Disabled people therefore rely heavily on council housing, and the policy of successive Conservative governments throughout the 1980s of seeking to reduce the public sector has had a tremendously damaging impact. Although councils have increased the proportion of new housing which is wheelchair accessible or adaptable, they are simply building far less housing, and much of the council housing stock has been sold under 'Right to Buy' policies.

The shrinking public housing sector has led to a sharp increase in the number of homeless people, with disabled people making up a large proportion.[22] In fact the homeless statistics greatly underestimate the extent of the problem. Jenny Morris points out:

Hidden homelessness is a real problem for people with disabilities who are unable to leave hospital, a long stay institution or a parental home, or who are imprisoned in an inaccessible home. A report by the Royal College of Physicians in 1986 estimated that well over half the physically disabled people under retirement age in residential/institutional care are in inappropriate places, such as geriatric hospital wards and old people's homes.[23]

Legal solutions
In its final form the Civil Rights Bill would have prohibited attitudinal prejudices and required those renting or selling property to make reasonable modifications in their practices. In this respect it is interesting to look at the American Federal Fair Housing Amendment Act 1988. This prohibits landlords from discriminating against disabled people (as well as prohibiting discrimination on the basis of race), and gives a non-exclusive list of activities which constitute discrimination. Landlords must allow disabled people to make 'reasonable modifica-

tions' to their units. However, these modifications must be at the tenants' expense. Landlords must also make 'reasonable accommodations' to their rules and services to allow disabled people equal opportunities to occupy their buildings. So, for example, where pets are banned occupants and visitors must still be allowed to use guide or signal dogs.

To have any effective impact on the lack of accessible housing an anti-discrimination law would, in addition, need to extend the Building Regulations to cover private housing. Thus, the Fair Housing Act imposes design requirements on new housing with four or more units. (These requirements are basically those for adaptable housing.) If the building has a lift all units are covered; if not, only the ground-floor units are covered.

The importance of effective enforcement was stressed by Adolf Ratzka in his discussion of the Swedish law at a conference organised by Shelter.[24] Swedish building codes, applying to all new multi-family housing built since 1977, require mobility standards of access, including lifts. (About half the Swedish population lives in multi-family accommodation.) Less stringent standards apply to single-family properties. Progress towards an accessible housing stock has been quite slow, partly due to a lack of new building.

Ratzka considers poor enforcement to be a critical weakness of Swedish laws: 'There is no evaluation of compliance with the access norms, but my hunch is that it's far from 100 per cent ... Swedish access norms are paper tigers without teeth.'[25] The responsibility for enforcement lies with the local government. Ratzka compares the situation to that in the United States, where a woman who had to be carried up two steps to get into a restaurant was awarded $70,000 from the restaurant owner, because it had undergone major remodelling and had to be fully accessible. 'As soon as the owners lost the case they made all other restaurants in the chain accessible.'[26]

The Codes have, nevertheless, achieved significant progress: by 1984 7 per cent of Stockholm's housing was wheelchair accessible. Ratzka comments: 'Seven percent may not sound much but it is noticeable. In Stockholm we do not experience the same difficulties in finding accessible housing as some of my friends do in other European cities.'[27]

Even this brief survey of the housing problems faced by disabled people should make it clear that merely enacting these measures would have a strictly limited impact. Although the changes in building requirements for new housing would have a gradual impact, they would need to be supplemented by adequate state funding for adaptation grants. Moreover, as long as public sector building is curtailed and disabled people are unable to afford private sector rents or mortgages, little will change. Improving the income position of disabled people would be the ideal solution, but in reality disabled people are likely to continue to have lower resources on average than able-bodied people.

To compensate for this, the system of distributing housing according to need must be strengthened through public sector provision. The homeless persons legislation is the only legally binding duty imposed on the state to provide housing; local housing authorities often have such limited resources that they are unable to help anyone who falls outside this legislative obligation.

The Housing Act 1985 imposes a duty on local authorities to provide accommodation for people who are homeless and in priority need (provided that they cannot be deemed to have made themselves homeless intentionally). Those in priority need include persons who are 'vulnerable as a result of old age, mental illness or handicap, physical disability' or with whom such a person resides.[28] A person will be deemed to be homeless even if s/he has accommodation if this is unsuitable for his/her needs. However, courts have interpreted this provision in such a way as to deny assistance to disabled people, even where they are living in situations which to any reasonable person would seem desperately unsuitable.

The most outrageous court decision with regard to local authorities' duties to house homeless disabled people was in a House of Lords case in 1993.[29] The case involved a Bangladeshi woman described by the report as lacking 'hearing, speech and education'. The local authority decided that she was 'so disabled that she could not make an application for housing'. This decision was upheld on the basis that a duty was owed only to those who had the capacity to understand and respond to such an offer, and local authorities have the power to evaluate a person's capacities subject to no appeal, save the (very limited) avenue of judicial review.

Crucial though the issues of increased state provision are, in the form of improved homelessness laws and adaptation grants, these cannot be addressed within an anti-discrimination framework. Such a law, by its very nature, focuses on providing equality between disabled and non-disabled people. But since able-bodied people do not have a right to decent housing, equality with them would not produce such a right for disabled people. Clearly, however, an anti-discriminatory perspective could be used to challenge and improve statutory provision, as has been the case for black people by the CRE. Local authorities should be banned from discriminating in service provision (in the way that they did towards the deaf Bangladeshi woman). However, a specific right to housing could not be inferred from anti-discrimination principles, any more than women or black people are accorded such rights to housing.

The provisions which impose a duty on local authorities to house the homeless must be strengthened and adequately funded as part of an anti-discrimination initiative. Specifically, the situation on hidden homelessness amongst disabled people needs to be recognised, so that institutions are seen as not constituting 'suitable housing'.

When arguing for such provision, it is important to look at the broader picture of costs. The reduced need for institutions produces substantial savings. Similarly, adaptations to private homes frequently enable disabled people to live more independently, requiring less help either from unpaid assistants or from state services. In addition, adaptations benefit more than the individual living in them at a particular time, as they increase the stock of accessible housing in society:

> Having access ... will not only allow people like me to move around more freely in order to pursue their education, find jobs, marry and raise families, but will make life easier for our older citizens as well. They will manage much easier in their homes and the need for services and institutions will be greatly reduced. In short everyone gains. This is true for accessibility in general in that building barrier-free benefits everyone.[30]

Transport

No effective legislative progress has been made in the area of entitlement to open access to transport systems. Some transport providers have been placed under a statutory duty to 'have regard to' the needs of disabled passengers, but in practice this is too generalised and weak a requirement to be capable of effecting significant change. Similarly, the Disabled Person's Transport Advisory Committee, established in 1985, is an advisory body with no power over the Department of Transport.

Some progress has been made, however. Ninety per cent of new trains in Britain have wide entry doors, and automatic doors with grab rails are now standard design features, as are spaces for wheelchairs in carriages. The first low floor buses, which can be used by people in wheelchairs, went on trial in 1994. Progress has also been made in some areas with wheelchair usable taxis. Over a quarter of London taxis are now accessible, but it will not be compulsory for all London cabs to be accessible until 2000. Outside London the picture is patchy. Local authorities are responsible for licensing taxis, and over 30 councils are insisting that cabs are accessible before a new licence is issued.

With urban transport systems the picture is again patchy. A very few systems, such as that in Tyne and Wear, were designed to be accessible for wheelchair users. In contrast, until September 1993 London Transport banned people in wheelchairs from using the underground system, except between a few ground-level stations, with prior notice.

Despite the lifting of the formal ban the reality remains that access to most parts of the system is appalling.

Progress has been painfully slow and even this is put in jeopardy by privatisation – for example, the proposed deregulation of taxis. The lack of any legislative backing for the principle of equal access makes any improvements fragile. The government's continued opposition to imposing meaningful access obligations on transport operators was made clear in the Railways Act 1993, which privatised the railways. The government resisted the amendment put forward by the disability lobby which would have required operators to provide access to disabled users, and substituted the feeble requirement that operators should 'have regard to' their needs.

A basic necessity such as transport should not depend upon the whim of local agencies. The technical facilities are available to make transport accessible to all. Equal access to transport should be regarded as a right, and a timetable for accessible transport established, as has been done under the ADA.

Primary and secondary education

The practices which we described in Chapter 1 as typifying the way in which the welfare state treated 'disabled' people (segregation, medicalisation and exclusion) have been very powerful in education. The Education Act 1944, which established a national system of free education for the first time, strengthened pre-existing policies on segregation. Local education authorities were required to make separate provision for disabled children, and a set of medical categories such as epileptic, delicate and educationally sub-normal were established. Until the Education (Handicapped Children) Act 1970 a substantial number of children were still being denied any access to education on the basis that they were too disabled to benefit.

The framework for current educational provision for disabled children was established by the Education Act 1981. Although the Education Act 1993 repeals and replaces most of the 1981 Act, and institutes major changes in mainstream education provision, the basic framework for 'special' children remains unchanged.

The 1981 Act, and the Warnock Report from which it derived, have been cast as milestones in the education of disabled children, in that they abolished medical categories and placed increased emphasis on integration. Other commentators have stressed the continuities with the past contained in these two documents.[31] In part, these diverging assessments stem from ambiguities in the texts. At one point the Report makes clear that special educational needs are relative, and that the distinction between 'two types of children, the handicapped and the non-handicapped' is a false one, created by the school system:

Whether a disability or significant difficulty constitutes an educational handicap for an individual child, and if so to what extent, will depend upon a variety of factors. Schools differ, often widely, in outlook, expertise, resources, accommodation, organisation and physical and social surroundings, all of which help determine the degree to which the individual is educationally handicapped ... It is thus impossible to establish precise criteria for defining what constitutes handicap.[32]

However, the general tenor of the report is permeated with 'the themes of guilt, suffering [and] burden'.[33] Bureaucratic professionalism is still firmly in control, while the new discourse of rights is only feebly present in the Report and Act; it was introduced but not provided with any practical means to put it into effect.

Resources

The 1981 law potentially serves two purposes. First it provides, in a loose sense, a right to resources. Children with special needs have the right to have those special needs catered for. The instrument through which this right is enforced is a statement of special needs drawn up by the local authority. LEAs have a duty to identify, assess and provide for the children who have significantly greater learning difficulties than the majority of children of the same age, or whose impairments prevent them from using mainstream provision.[34]

Authorities are to judge on a 'professional' basis what form of education is appropriate for these children. Parents may request an assessment if they consider that their child has special educational needs.[35] Alternatively, LEAs may initiate the assessment process. A formal assessment may result in a Statement of Special Educational Needs (SEN),[36] describing a child's particular needs and how they should be met. During this process, the professionals must consult parents, but their wishes need not be followed. Children's feelings should be 'considered'.

Fulcher's assessment is that the radical potential of the Act is severely limited: 'Despite wide interpretation that the 1981 Act confers new rights on parents whose child is deemed to have special educational needs, it is clear that the Act retains the language, hierarchy and politics of professionalism.'[37] A shortage of resources has ironically meant that this professionalism has been used to legitimise a rationing system and constrain protest. The CORAD Report's comments on the Act are somewhat more blunt:

... the Education Act does little to improve the current situation of disabled children. It will still be a matter for the Education Authority to decide where to educate the disabled child and the Act does nothing to oblige Authorities to develop a greater range of facilities for disabled children in ordinary schools.[38]

The lack of an independent appeals system for parents has allowed this process to go largely unchecked. Under the 1981 Act there is no provision for appeals outside the educational apparatus, although the Education Act 1993 has now remedied this by providing for independent tribunals. The Act, and its accompanying Code of Practice,[39] also contain criteria for establishing when assessments and statements are required, what their contents should be, and a timetable for their production. However, whilst these procedural changes impose valuable restrictions on LEAs, the fundamental approach remains unchanged.

Integration

The second ostensible purpose of the 1981 Act was to counteract the historical segregation of disabled children. A major barrier to the integration of disabled children is the physical inaccessibility of many school buildings. The CSDPA stated that all new school buildings had to be accessible where 'reasonable and practicable'. This has had little impact, mainly because few schools have been built since it came into force.

On the subject of integration, Warnock herself comments: 'People say we fudged integration, but we fudged it as a matter of policy.'[40] The failure of the Education Act 1981 to produce integration is therefore not surprising. Thus, whilst the Act endorses the general principle of integration, it has huge loopholes. Integration is permissible as long as it meets the educational needs of the child and is compatible with the 'provision of efficient education for the children with whom he will be educated' and 'the efficient use of resources'.[41]

The Act has had little impact on the powerful trends towards segregation, with the percentage of children in special schools relative to the whole school population moving from 1.41 per cent in 1977 to 1.35 per cent in 1989.[42] The most comprehensive survey to date has found that 24 per cent of disabled children living at home go to 'special schools', with a further 10 per cent having another form of segregated 'special' provision.[43]

One of the justifications for segregation under the 1981 Act, and an excuse frequently resorted to in discussions of the feasibility of full integration, is the issue of cost. However, until recently no research had been conducted on this question. In 1992 the Spastics Society, in association with the National Union of Teachers, commissioned Coopers and Lybrand to research the costs of integrating physically disabled children into mainstream schooling.[44] On the basis of a survey of sample LEAs they concluded that the costs of further progressing integration were not particularly high, with the exception of the costs of premises' conversion and the transitional expenses.

A follow-up survey was carried out, examining the costs of converting school premises.[45] The conclusion was that:

> ... current accessibility to school premises can be significantly improved, to a level where: 75 per cent of the primary schools provide access to three-quarters or more of their teaching accommodation; 50 per cent of secondary schools provide access to all their teaching accommodation ... for an investment of ... c. £14 per primary pupil and £82 per secondary pupil.[46]

The issue of resources is crucial if disabled children are not to experience integration as providing a second-rate education. Colin Barnes clearly expresses the dangers of the situation: 'The rhetoric of integration could represent nothing more than a politically convenient ploy to reduce public expenditure ... Without a firm commitment to eradicate discrimination in all its forms within the mainstream sector ... these fears might well be justified.'[47]

Recent developments
The huge changes in the broader educational structure over the last five years have made these concerns even more pertinent. The Education Reform Act 1988 allows schools to opt out of LEA control and become self-governing, introduced a national curriculum and encourages competition between schools. Disabled children can be exempted completely from the requirements of the national curriculum, or it may be 'modified'. Schools are being forced to concentrate their staffing and funding policies on core curriculum subjects, and this has meant pressure to redirect priorities away from cross-curricular responsibilities such as special needs and pastoral care:[48]

> The Local Management of Schools – with the accompanying phenomena of opting out, the entrepreneurial culture, the publishing of exam results and the intensifying competitiveness of schools – does not serve the interests of any children, and is certainly detrimental to promoting greater inclusion in mainstream schools of children with special needs.[49]

The Education Act 1993 accentuates this marginalisation by transferring the role of LEAs to a new central government-appointed Funding Agency for Schools. LEAs, however, are expected to retain responsibility for special educational needs.

Legal solutions
It might be thought that with such an array of provision already in place, a new law in this area might be superfluous, or add needless

complexity. On the contrary, the Civil Rights (Disabled Persons) Bill would have provided an orienting, non-discriminatory framework into which all existing educational provision would have had to fit. This would have applied to both public and private provision (whereas existing law merely imposes obligations on the state), and to schools, LEAs, universities, central government and quangos such as the Further Education Funding Council (FEFC). We have already seen that this has proved useful in the areas of sex and race discrimination.

The Bill would also at last have initiated significant progress towards integration, by requiring educational institutions to make modifications to their premises and service delivery (for example, by providing support services or exams in alternative formats). However, rather than leaving the degree and nature of such modifications to be determined by a case by case approach, regulations and a Code of Practice could usefully establish the responsibilities of the relevant authorities in this area.

It would, of course, be important to be precise about the impact of an anti-discrimination law on the existing framework for 'special needs' provision. In particular, it would be helpful to expand and clarify the provisions for integration. The Education Act 1993 should be modified in line with the amendments which the Centre for Studies on Integration in Education attempted to introduce when the Bill was originally before Parliament. These proposals would have made it more difficult to place disabled children in segregated schools. An LEA could only have insisted on such a placement if there was compelling evidence that the child's educational needs could not be met in a mainstream school even if provided with adequate support services, or if the child's behaviour was likely to be 'seriously detrimental' to the welfare of others in the school. This proposal would have allowed a six-year lead-in period and required LEAs to draw up integration plans. Back in 1982, the CORAD Report recommended that LEAs should be required to draw up such plans, and should have a duty to render as many mainstream schools as possible accessible to disabled children and adults, making the point that access might equally be required by disabled parents, employees or governors.[50] In addition, there is a need for a national integration policy and for guidance from central government on how to implement the integration clause, requiring the monitoring of its effects.

The issue of parental choice is at the centre of current government thinking on education. It is significant that the 1993 Act gives a veto to parents who want their child to go to a special school, but does not provide the same veto for parents wishing their child to experience an integrated education. There may be occasions in which disabled children and their families prefer segregated provision. The most compelling example is the case of deaf children who may wish to be able to socialise with other children who share their primary language – sign. However, in all cases, for choice to be meaningful it must be within the context of adequate resources and a genuinely welcoming atmosphere within schools. The last point requires the adoption and implementation of anti-discrimination policies within schools and training for teachers. Although still inadequate, these types of provision have been encouraged by the sex and race laws.

Finally, it is important to bear in mind that an anti-discrimination law will be the starting point in a process of struggle to secure equal and adequate education for all disabled children. 'A new law may be seen as just one significant event in the general process of service and policy development.'[51]

Further and higher education

The shortage of information about the situation of disabled people in further and higher education is testimony to the low priority accorded to this issue. Recent research estimates that only 0.3 per cent of the student population in polytechnics and universities is disabled.[52] On the supply side, more than a fifth of colleges in a 1987 survey reported that they might have to reject a disabled applicant because of poor access or inadequate support.[53] Half of them reported that their teaching blocks were inaccessible, less than a quarter supported visually impaired students on mainstream courses, and under a third provided assistance to hearing impaired students.

The Further and Higher Education Act 1992 has transferred responsibility for most further education (FE) courses from LEAs to the Further Education Funding Council. The one hope for slight improvement in the present situation is that the FEFC has ringfenced funding to enable colleges to become more accessible and has invited applications from colleges.

If the Civil Rights (Disabled Persons Bill) had been passed it would have outlawed discrimination from the application processes, and required modifications to be provided both to physical access and to the delivery of teaching, along the same lines as schools.

As with school-age education, it would be valuable to supplement this broad framework with a detailed national plan for improving access, and with regulations establishing what support services institutions would be obliged to provide. The regulations established under Section 504 of the US Rehabilitation Act could provide useful guidance. An important element of these regulations is that they require all publicly funded institutions to carry out access audits and evaluate their systems generally to determine the extent to which they incorporate the maximum accessibility to disabled people.

Employment

Since the Civil Rights (Disabled Persons) Bill closely followed the provisions of the ADA in the area of employment, the consequences of introducing such a law will already be clear from previous chapters. It may, however, be worth emphasising again the importance of moving beyond the approach of the sex and race laws in this area. Unless anti-discrimination legislation requires employers to make some alterations to work structures, disabled people will continue to be confined to the inferior jobs in which they have traditionally been employed, since the other jobs have been structured in such a way that they exclude the broad range of abilities which disabled people represent. If legislation merely addresses discriminatory attitudes it will therefore serve to perpetuate past discrimination.

As the account of the genesis of anti-discrimination legislation for people with disabilities reveals, the issue of the potential costs involved in integrating disabled people into the economy has been the focus of opposition to the legislation. Proponents of the legislation cite studies which show that the average price of accommodations is low. For example, a 1982 study[54] showed that over half of accommodations provided by federal contractors under the Rehabilitation Act were simple and could be provided at no extra cost, and 30 per cent of those accommodations which did impose costs required expenditures of under $500 dollars. Only 8 per cent involved costs over $2,000. In fact, only 22 per cent of disabled workers were reported as requiring any accommodation. Such arguments are a two-edged sword in that, while assisting the passing of legislation and countering stereotypes, they may also be used to limit the extent of accommodations which are legally required, so that those jobs which require more extensive alterations remain closed to disabled people.

The rest of this section will examine the adequacy of existing provision in this area in Britain, considering whether aspects of it might usefully be retained within an anti-discriminatory framework.

Quota scheme

The only law which specifically addresses the issue of the employment of disabled people is the Disabled Persons (Employment) Act 1944. This requires employers of 20 or more people to employ a minimum of 3 per cent registered disabled people. Strictly speaking it is not an offence for covered employers to employ less than this quota, but they commit an offence if they are under quota and employ a non-registered disabled person unless they have a permit.[55] Such permits can be issued by the Department of Employment on the basis that there are no suitable registered disabled candidates for the post. The 1944 Act makes it an offence for employers of 20 or more people to dismiss a registered disabled person without reasonable cause, if by doing so they will employ less than their 3 per cent quota.[56] No definition of 'reasonable cause' is provided, and the absence of prosecutions has prevented the development of one through case law.

In practice, the Act is widely flouted, with 80 per cent of employers failing to meet their quota and permits being handed out en masse. The major reason for this is that prosecutions can only be brought by (or with the consent of) the Secretary of State for Employment, and there has been a reluctance to enforce the Act. Only ten prosecutions have ever been brought, none since 1975.

Disability groups have called for the enforcement of the quota scheme. But even if the Act were to be effectively enforced it would not fulfil the need for legal protection against discrimination. It does not ban discrimination against disabled people. Many employers are not covered, and even those who are can comply with their duties by employing disabled people at the lowest grades in their organisation, paying them discriminatory wages and depriving them of any opportunity for promotion. Indeed this is not far from the truth of the present situation.

Although not adequate in itself, if anti-discrimination legislation was passed a suitably modified quota scheme, or alternative form of positive action, would provide a much needed supplement. Previous chapters have stressed the importance of positive action, in the form of monitoring the composition of the workforce and, where necessary, setting percentage goals. It is ironic that in Britain, whilst quotas remain anathema in the areas of sex and race, they exist in the area of disability. It would be wise to retain the principle established by disability quotas, even once anti-discrimination legislation for disabled people was in place.

However, the quota scheme in its present form cannot fulfil this role because it is fatally weakened by its origins in a welfarist response to disability, rather than a rights discourse. Crucially, in order to count as disabled it is necessary to register as such, and a person must be 'substantially handicapped in obtaining or retaining employment'.[57] This definition seems to imply that registered disabled workers are less capable, and people have not surprisingly been reluctant to stigmatise themselves in this way. At the same time, if a quota system is to provide a useful supplement to anti-discrimination legislation it will need to ensure that employers do not seek to comply by employing those with the 'easiest' disabilities to accommodate. It may well be necessary to narrow the focus to specific forms of disability (as do the Federal government quotas mentioned in Chapter 4), or perhaps specify that a certain percentage of the workforce must have required reasonable accommodation. Alternatively, as in some European countries, people who are eligible for state disability benefits could be counted towards the quota.

Unfair dismissal

Although the 1944 quota scheme is the only law specifically targeted at disabled workers, they are also covered by the general laws regulating employment. Of these the most significant is the law protecting employees against unfair dismissal (Employment Protection Consolidation Act 1978). This law is enforceable by individuals through the same network of industrial tribunals as the employment sections of the race and sex legislation. There are major limitations on the scope of this protection – notably the fact that it only applies to long-term employees (two years full-time or five years part-time), and that it only regulates dismissals. Nevertheless, it is interesting to look at the case law, both to establish the limitations of the current approach and also because it will indicate the attitude of the tribunals and judges who will be responsible for adjudicating any anti-discrimination law.

The guidelines which employers can derive from the case law are vague and contradictory. The most worrying series of cases are those in which the tribunal refuses to defend a worker against an employer's mistaken assumptions about his/her abilities. For example, in a case concerning the effect on a man's work-capacity of his epileptic seizures the tribunal stated:

> Obviously an employer cannot claim that a reason for dismissal is substantial if it is a whimsical or capricious reason which no person with ordinary sense would entertain. But ... where the belief is one which is genuinely held, and particularly is one which most employers would be expected to adopt, it may be a substantial reason even where modern sophisticated opinion can be adduced to suggest that it has no scientific foundation.[58]

Fortunately, there is a contradictory strand of cases which holds that an employer is required to consult with the employee and seek appropriate advice about any 'medical' problems. In another case a man with symptoms similar to epilepsy, was dismissed because his co-workers were unwilling to work with him. In this instance his dismissal was held to be unfair because his employer made no attempt to find out the medical position or discuss this with the co-workers.[59]

In general terms, the requirement is that disabled employees (particularly when they are 'registered' and where this fact is known to the employer) are entitled to 'extra consideration'. Unfortunately, this is so vague that it amounts to legitimating the whims of tribunal members. The leading case gives a clear illustration of how paternalistic this approach can be:

> An employer ... has to ... say 'I must watch this, because I am not allowed to discontinue this employment unless I have reasonable

cause to do so. It won't do simply to say he did not put up an adequate performance in the capability stakes. I have got to assess his personal position.' It may well be that if an employer reminds himself of that fact, he may well say 'We are so sorry for this fellow, we will not even put him at risk.' A reasonable employer is entitled to take that view. At the other end of the scale, a reasonable employer would be entitled to take the view 'I am very sorry for this chap, but he really is absolutely hopeless. We have tried desperately hard with him and, having considered ... that his employment must not be discontinued without reasonable cause, we have plenty of reasonable cause because the chap is just not up to it.'[60]

There is clearly no understanding here of the processes of discrimination operating against disabled people. However, it is possible to glimpse a trace of a logical framework within most of the cases. Interestingly enough, the commonest approach is to balance the interest of the individual disabled person against the cost that this imposes on employers. For example, cases have held that employers with workers whose disabilities result in increased levels of absence should provide posts where such absences can be absorbed without due disruption;[61] that they should be flexible in their work requirements and investigate alternative work arrangements including part-time work[62] and alternative means of carrying out the work tasks.[63]

This is broadly similar to the reasonable accommodation approach in the Americans with Disabilities Act. This is not to say that the existing framework as set out in the unfair dismissal law is satisfactory. In the absence of specific provision, tribunals are unwilling to impose any significant requirements on employers. Moreover, 'extra consideration' is understood as a charitable gesture, rather than as a non-discriminatory mode of operating. Disabled employees are presented with the classic choice between asking that their disability is ignored, and asking for paternalistic favours.

The case law also makes it clear that tribunals and judges will need extensive disability equality training if they are to prove capable of implementing an anti-discrimination law. A greater representation of disabled people on the tribunals is also important. As we have seen, these issues have also been highlighted in the sex and race laws, and an additional proposal is that a specialist 'equality' tribunal be established to adjudicate such cases.

Sheltered employment – can it be retained within the anti-discriminatory framework?

The oldest form of specialist provision for the employment of disabled people is sheltered workshops. Charitable foundations provided a number of segregated employment establishments for disabled people from the late nineteenth century onwards, with local authorities following from the beginning of the twentieth century. Central government funding for such schemes was provided in the Disabled Persons (Employment) Acts of 1944 and 1958. Currently approximately 14,000 people are employed in such institutions.

The work in such organisations has traditionally been unskilled and manual, and the managerial positions are almost entirely occupied by able-bodied employees. The wages are desperately low. The rationale for such institutions is that the disabled persons employed within them are not capable of functioning within 'open' employment.

Sheltered workshops, as they have traditionally been run, are in any event out of favour. It is recognised that they ghettoise disabled workers and restrict their employment opportunities. In recent years a new, more integrated form of sheltered employment has been introduced – the sheltered placement scheme (SPS). In essence this operates to subsidise disabled employees who have been classified as less than 80 per cent productive in open employment. There are currently approximately 6,000 workers on SPSs.

Despite the integrationist approach of such schemes, there would be problems locating them within a non-discriminatory framework. At present funding limitations restrict SPS places to low-paid jobs and as such place a brake on career development for disabled workers. More fundamentally, the rationale behind SPS is the medical model of disability. The danger is that such a scheme perpetuates the stereotype of disabled workers as less productive and becomes an easy option for employers. Take the following example: a teacher in a comprehensive school loses most of her hearing. She can still teach, but has discipline problems with her unruly class. This problem could be resolved in a number of ways. The teacher could take medical retirement on the basis that she is no longer fit for work, the school could employ an assistant either from its own funds or by using subsidised employment, classes could be swapped to secure a less unruly class, or a place on SPS could be applied for.

Collectivist supplements

Nevertheless, the SPS scheme could be incorporated within a framework which recognised discrimination as the central problem faced by disabled people, provided it was understood as state assistance to employers where reasonable accommodation was unable to bring disabled people up to full productivity. There is a need for a broad range of government assistance to employers to enable them to meet the additional needs of disabled employees. This would reduce the costs of individual employers, recognising that the legacy of excluding disabled people from the workforce is a social problem which needs to be addressed through collective action. The American experience shows that courts will be more willing to order extensive accommodations where the costs for these is not imposed on the individual employer, but met on a social basis.

The framework already exists in Britain for this collectivist supplement to the anti-discrimination framework. A variety of state assistance is available to employers of disabled people. Launched in 1994, the Access to Work programme, an expanded version of old schemes, provides a wide range of support that includes payments for interpreters for deaf people and personal assistants for some physically disabled people.

The existence of this programme means that were anti-discrimination legislation to be introduced employers would be unable to use cost as an excuse for continuing to exclude disabled workers. This would represent an improvement on the position in America, where such a broad range of state assistance for disabled workers is not available, although some support, including tax credits where businesses incur disability related expenses, is provided.

Disability leave

Most disabled people are not born with an impairment but acquire one during the course of their lives. People who are born with an impairment or acquire one at an early age are more likely to participate in the workforce than people who become disabled at a later age. Research by Social and Community Planning Research (SCPR) has found that 65 per cent of workers who became disabled left their employers.[64] People who become disabled are likely to underestimate their own abilities to continue working, particularly as employers, doctors and other 'professionals' are likely to reinforce the attitude that disability inevitably excludes a person from the workforce. In some instances adaptations to the work environment will be required, in others the disabled person needs a chance to acquire new skills to adapt to his or her new situation.

The commonest response to disability is medical retirement. The concept of disability leave is currently being piloted by a number of employers so that they can keep their disabled staff. Under the scheme, an employee who becomes disabled will be allowed time off to retrain or to give the employer time to adapt the work environment. If the pilot is successful, the government will be pressed to place disability leave on the statute books. This would be another useful supplement to the ADA, under which law an individual is allowed time off depending on the outcome of an assessment as to whether an accommodation is 'reasonable'.

Advice services

To provide advice for newly disabled people and their employers, and to operate the government assistance schemes effectively, requires a network of disability and employment advisers. The lack of adequate information and advice has been pinpointed as one of the weaknesses of the ADA in operation.[65] At present, a network of civil servants with precisely this remit does exist in Britain. However, the Disability Employment Advisers, who operate from Job Centres, are notoriously under-skilled and many appear to share disablist prejudices.[66] More disabled people need to be recruited into these posts and equipped with adequate training.

State benefits

Any government is likely to insist that the social security system is exempt from the provisions of an anti-discrimination law, as we have seen in the context of sex discrimination law. Nevertheless, once such legislation is passed it will shift the terms of the debate from the charitable welfarist model, described in Chapter 1, to one based on rights, equality and entitlements. In so doing it will provide valuable ammunition for those seeking to remodel the welfare state along more progressive lines, and I touch on some of these issues later in this section.

However, there are also dangers associated with the move away from the welfarist mode. In the current British climate of cuts in welfare expenditure, there is a real danger that arguments and actions which focus on bringing disabled people into the workforce will be used as a justification for withdrawing or cutting payments to them. Paradoxically, one of the most significant barriers to disabled people entering the workforce is the structure of the welfare benefits system. I will therefore explore how disabled people's need for additional resources in order to live independently might be met without jeopardising their ability to enter the labour force, before considering the broader issue of how the state should meet the additional costs of disability.

Exclusion from the labour market

Many disabled people rely on the basic income maintenance benefit in the British welfare system, Income Support. In order to qualify for disability-specific income maintenance benefits (Severe Disablement Allowance or Invalidity Benefit [IVB]) claimants must establish that they are 'incapable' of work.

Many disabilities impede the ability to work full-time or fluctuate over time. Part-time work has become more available than it used to be, but generally entails poorer wages, work conditions and job security.[67] Women tend to be concentrated in part-time work and disabled women are therefore particularly likely to seek this. An important goal must be to improve conditions for part-time workers.

Moreover, the state benefit system makes it very difficult for disabled people to work part-time without suffering great income loss. For many years disability groups have campaigned for a partial incapacity allowance,[68] and it was claimed that the Disability Working Allowance (DWA), introduced in 1992, would meet this need. It has, however, proved to be a resounding failure. By October 1992 successful claims numbered only 2,401, just 11 per cent of applications received.[69] The two major reasons for claims being rejected were that the applicants worked too few hours to qualify (less than 16 hours a week), or did not already have a job. (It is necessary already to have started work before claiming.) The tight means test is very complex, and frequently means that a person will be worse off on DWA unless he or she is on very low wages. Welfare rights advisers in a 1992 survey believed that 'the benefit levels were an insult.'[70]

The Royal Association for Disability and Rehabilitation (RADAR)[71] has argued instead for a simple system which would pay a proportion of Invalidity Benefit for the proportion of the week for which a disabled person was unable to work.[72]

Growth in numbers of disability claimants

The tendency of workers who become disabled to take early retirement has increased the numbers of people claiming state disability benefits, particularly Invalidity Benefit. The numbers of people claiming 'incapacity' benefits rose between 1970 and 1991 in the United States, Sweden, Germany, Great Britain, Ireland and Australia.[73] The British government has chosen to tackle this issue by seeking to restrict the eligibility conditions (in effect penalising disabled individuals) rather than by looking at the broader causes of the increase and attacking it at source.

The rise in the numbers of IVB claimants is not due primarily to an increasing number of new claimants. Research by the Policy Studies Institute calculates that only a third of the increase was the result of new claimants. This in turn was a product of the ageing population and the increasing number of women entering the labour market and hence becoming eligible for IVB.[74] The major factor in the increase of IVB claimants is the decrease in the numbers of people coming off IVB and obtaining work:

> What seems to have happened is that there has been a fairly constant number of people leaving work on health grounds over the years. But as the labour market has tightened, they have found it more and more difficult to get back into work ... This explanation for the increasing cost of IVB lies in the economy as a whole, and in the hiring and firing of employees, rather than in a change in the behaviour of individual claimants.[75]

A survey of recipients by the Department of Social Security in 1993 found that four-fifths of people receiving IVB did not expect to work again.[76] Severity of disability and amount of time on IVB affected the likelihood that claimants were still hoping to work. This suggests that disabled people, particularly older and severely disabled people, frequently become discouraged from seeking work. The attitudes of those still seeking work are an important indication of the reason for this discouragement: they had low expectations of their future salary, and their confidence in their ability to work limited their search. The availability of work suitable to their health and employers' attitudes were also important factors in limiting their employment chances. This suggests that a more progressive response to the increasing numbers of disabled people who are dependent on state benefits would be to tackle employer discrimination and provide retraining where required, as well as skilled employment advice.

We have seen that the prospect of reducing the 'welfare dependency' of disabled people was a major factor behind the decision of the American government to support the ADA. It is also an important argument for the British disability movement.

Care must be taken, however, that such arguments are not used to restrict access to welfare benefits for those who need them. Work commonly extracts higher demands on the lives of disabled people. Probably the majority of disabled people would choose to pay this additional price; others may not feel able to do so. Two people with identical disabilities and jobs might choose differently. This would be 'choice' of a completely different nature from that faced by an able-bodied person. It is more comparable to the choice of a person over the state retirement age to continue working. Indeed, the situation of disabled people in this respect parallels that of older people, and of course there is a considerable overlap.[77]

There is increasing pressure from groups representing older people for discrimination against older people to be made illegal. Undoubtedly the large numbers of older disabled people who stop looking for work experience discrimination on grounds of both age and disability. However, there is a danger that the argument that older workers are good workers could be used to push up the state retirement age (and there is a drive to do this as a further cost-cutting measure in many European countries).

For both disabled and older workers the choice of whether or not to work should be made available through anti-discrimination legislation, without penalising those who choose not to work. They have earned this right. The conflict between distribution by need and by waged labour makes this a difficult goal to achieve, but nevertheless an essential one.

Extra costs of disability

Disabled people incur a broad range of additional costs, not least the cost of personal assistance. Some additional expenses arise from the inaccessibility of the environment – for example, the costs of travel when public transport is inaccessible, or the costs of residential care.

The social security provision for disabled people is extremely complicated, discriminatory between different groups of disabled people (1991 figures from Disability Alliance showed the gap in benefit between two similarly disabled people could be as much as £247.95 per week)[78] and grossly inadequate. A Disability Income Group study has found an additional financial expenditure of an average of £69.92 per week was incurred on account of impairment.[79]

The goal for the disability movement is a comprehensive disability income. The Disability Alliance proposes that such a scheme should consist of two components. A disablement allowance would be payable to meet the extra costs of disability, solely on the basis of the restrictions imposed on an individual's activities. A disablement *pension* would be payable to anyone excluded from the labour market on the basis of their disability. This would include recognition that many disabled people would be available only for part-time work.

At present, these needs are met from a number of different state funding systems: local authority social services, the welfare benefits system and the Independent Living Fund, to name the three most important. These services should be provided so as not to rob disabled people of the opportunity to engage in the waged labour market. This means they need to be provided without charge to the individual, regardless of income, or with a substantial subsidy to prevent recipients being caught in a trap which means that they cannot afford to work.

The quality and control of these services are also crucial. The 'new era' of community care, introduced in April 1993 when the Community Care Act 1990 came into force, was less of a revolution than a technocratic reshuffling of inadequate resources. The stated intention was to shift the balance of finance away from residential care. However, too often the appropriate housing and financial resources required for independent living are simply not there.

There is no pretence that the aim is independent living. This is a fundamentally different concept expounded by the Independent Living Movement, with centres around the country. The key to independent living is that disabled individuals are given control over their own lives. Independent Living Centres set up alternative kinds of service provision run by disabled people themselves.

The issue of an adequate level of resources interconnects with the key issue of control. The concept of need remains central to the community care reforms and professionals continue to have the power to define and 'assess' disabled people's needs. Since this process takes place in the context of fixed budgets, there is a clear danger that financial limitations, rather than the needs of the disabled individual, will determine the assessment. The problem of unmet need is thus defined away, since the need does not officially exist unless it is recognised through an assessment process.

Two complementary solutions arise from the above argument. The first is the classic approach of welfare rights lobbyists: to reduce the element of discretion placed in the hands of state bureaucrats, by providing detailed specifications of entitlements, strict timetables and independent appeals procedures, preferably with access to legal advice. The second seeks to wrest power from state-paid professionals and put it in the hands of disabled people.

The present system's emphasis on need harks back to the post-war paternalist approach to welfare, whereas in other areas the Conservatives have been eager to replace this with a rhetoric of choice. Often the choices proffered by Conservatives have been illusory, because they have masked a failure to provide the resources required to make them meaningful. However, the concept does add an important dimension to the welfare system, provided there are guarantees that they will be backed by the necessary resources.

The system of assistance provided by local authority social services generally fails to offer even the most basic of choices, such as when to go to bed or to eat. The disability movement is asking for disabled people to be given the choice of arranging their own care, paid for by grants from local authorities. However, the government has declared that the National Assistance Act 1948 made such payments illegal, and opposed a Private Members Bill in 1993 which would have legalised such payments.[80] To understand its reasons we must look beyond the issue of resources, since direct payments have been found to be cost effective.[81] To an extent the government's resistance can be explained by its prejudiced views of the dependence of disabled people. However, it also touches on the fundamental issue of control and power. If disabled people have the power to determine their own care needs, why should professionals assess them? And professionals have provided a vital function to the state as the gate-keepers, or more accurately bouncers, of state services.

Necessary supplements

The Chronically Sick and Disabled Persons Act 1970 recognised for the first time two crucial issues for disabled people: the importance of information and consultation. However, as with its other provisions, these issues were only inadequately addressed.

Information
Disabled people are in general poorly informed about the services and the equipment available to them. The situation is not helped by the

complexity of provision and the professionalisation of services. The 1970 Act contains a requirement that local authorities publicise their services to disabled people.[82] This was later reinforced by Section 9 of the Disabled Persons (Services, Consultation and Representation) Act 1986. The principle is a vitally important one, since the impact of any legislation depends on people knowing about it.

This provision, however, has been widely ignored and has produced little of value. A Department of Health and Social Services Inspectorate report concluded: 'It was so discouraging that so little had been done by social services departments to provide relevant information in suitable formats for disabled people.'[83]

Similar difficulties have arisen with the Education Act 1981, because parents have not been given adequate information about the complicated statementing and assessment procedures to which their child may be subjected. Despite statutory requirements,[84] and DES guidance[85] setting out precisely what information LEAs should publish, there is substantial evidence that many fail to provide it.[86] One extensive survey commissioned by the government found that only 22 per cent of the parents of disabled children had heard of the assessment and statementing process.[87]

Access to the legal system

Chapter 6 discussed, in the context of the sex and race laws, the importance of subsidised access to legal advice and representation. This issue has become even more vital with the severe restrictions on financial eligibility for legal aid imposed in 1992. For any law to be effective, those whom it is designed to protect must have meaningful access to the legal system, and this requires a realistic level of state subsidy towards the cost of legal representation.

Disabled people have an additional hurdle to cross in using the legal system. Many courtrooms remain physically inaccessible, deaf people are not always provided with free sign language interpreters, nor are induction loops installed or information made available by tape or in braille for blind people. The Royal Commission on Criminal Justice has recommended a series of improvements, which are required to make the system accessible to disabled users.[88]

Consultation

An input into the policy making process is clearly vital to any disadvantaged group. Again the 1970 Act marks the first, tentative recognition of the importance of involving disabled people in the planning and running of services for their benefit. Sections 9 to 15 stressed the 'desirability' of the inclusion of people with experience of working with disabled persons, and in particular that such experts should themselves be disabled. In legal terms merely requiring authorities to 'have regard to the desirability' of something is extremely weak. Nevertheless, the principle was established.

Further progress in this area appeared to have been made with the Disabled Persons (Services, Consultation and Representation) Act 1986. Section 10 required local authorities to coopt people with specialist knowledge of disability to council committees. The same DSS report found that many local authorities had failed adequately to implement this section.[89]

The Community Care Act also includes a requirement for consultation. However, the existence of adequately funded groups of disabled people, both at a local and a national level, is a prerequisite for both the dissemination of information and effective consultation. There has been a burgeoning of self-help and advocacy groups of disabled people in the last ten years, but this is in spite of a severe shortage of funds, and resources are tightly stretched. Nevertheless, as we shall see in Chapter 8, it is the emergence of a national Disability Movement which has succeeded in putting anti-discrimination legislation firmly on the agenda.

Conclusion

This chapter has illustrated the complexity and inadequacy of the present legislation governing the lives of disabled people, and examined how these might be simplified within the framework of comprehensive anti-discrimination legislation. It has attempted to take a realistic view about what can and cannot be addressed within such a law. Even if such a law cannot address all the problems faced by disabled people, particularly those arising out of the lack of entitlement to resources (whether in state benefits, education or housing), it can fundamentally change the context in which all state policies will be viewed and implemented.

The present system is described by one critic as 'unworkable, untenable, disjointed and unenforceable',[90] to which could perhaps be added 'unaccountable and philosophically incoherent'. In contrast, the introduction of an overarching anti-discrimination statute would give clear guidelines for the development of policy and for the implementation of legislation. Similarly, the establishment of a Disablement Commission could incorporate the numerous bodies which currently exist to advise government on disability policy, as well as providing a crucial source of new guidance and strategic enforcement.

8
The Prospects for Disability Rights in Britain

The survey of the British law on disability in Chapter 7 gives a clear indication of how far short it falls in providing an adequate legislative protection against discrimination. Whilst the Chronically Sick and Disabled Persons Act 1970 and Education Act 1981, through their emphasis on desegregation and removing environmental barriers, represent real progress, their bureaucratic approach drastically limited their capacity to institute real change. Scotch characterises this approach as: 'The establishment of a symbolic right to access without substantive guarantees'.[1] This chapter outlines the development within Britain of a campaign for effective anti-discrimination legislation, and assesses its chances of success.

Growth of the disability movement

Undoubtedly, in Britain as in America, the key factor in fuelling the campaign for civil rights legislation for disabled people has been the growth of collective self-organisation by disabled people – the emergence and increasing militance of a disability movement. Organisations of disabled people have a long history in Britain, starting with the National League of the Blind and the British Deaf Association in the 1890s.

In the contemporary era the focus of campaigning was initially the goal of achieving adequate state benefits for disabled people. The 1960s saw the formation of the Disablement Income Group, followed in 1975 by the Disability Alliance. These groups tended to follow the model of conventional pressure groups, collecting information and lobbying governments for change on this basis.

However, since the mid-1970s a large number of organisations of disabled people with a more radical approach have been formed. Many of these were formed as self-help groups, to deal with the difficulties presented by both the able-bodied environment and the institutions of the welfare state (which in theory exist to serve disabled people, but as we have seen frequently represent some of the most significant barriers). A particular response to this failure of the state apparatus was

159

the creation of a network of Independent Living Centres, modelled on those set up in the United States.

As these groups have developed, they have increasingly devoted their attention to attempting to change the system while assisting their members to battle with the day to day consequences of discrimination and paternalist provision. The formation in 1981 of an umbrella organisation of such activist groups of disabled people, the British Council of Organisations of Disabled People (BCODP), undoubtedly represented a significant step in the emergence of a British 'disability movement'. The BCODP represents 80 organisations of disabled people and some 200,000 disabled individuals:

> The move towards self-organisation has prompted increasing numbers of disabled people to adopt a shared political identity, which in turn has helped build a new mood of confidence. Disabled people no longer ask for change but demand it. They are prepared to use a whole range of tactics in pursuit of their demands, including direct action and civil disobedience. It is because of this growing self-confidence that disabled people are forcing the issue of institutional discrimination onto the political agenda.[2]

Towards end of the 1980s this movement began to adopt radical strategies such as sit-ins and street demonstrations which we have already seen were used with such success by the American disability movement. They were found protesting against the degrading images of the Telethon fund-raising TV programme, blocking Oxford Street to highlight the inaccessible transport system, chaining themselves to railings to protest against the rejection of yet another anti-discrimination bill, or picketing the election campaign of the Conservative MP who had 'talked out' the Civil Rights Bill.

These actions are crucial for projecting an image of disabled people as dynamic participants in society, for educating the public and for promoting the need to reverse the discriminatory processes of society. Towards the end of 1993, the *New Statesman* could report that the Direct Action Network had a national register of more than a thousand disability activists willing to take part in civil disobedience.[3]

A development which may in the long run prove as significant is disabled people's increasing willingness to use the law, however imperfect in its present form. Through judicial reviews of state actions, claims against local authorities for breaches of contract and complaints to ombudsmen, disabled people have been actively challenging the discretionary nature of social services and educational provision. In 1993, for example, the local government ombudsman recommended that a local authority which had delayed more than three years in finding an appropriate educational placement for a boy with learning difficulties should pay £12,500.[4] At the same time, another council was ordered to pay £2,000 for excessive delay in providing adaptations for a house under Section 2 of the Chronically Sick and Disabled Persons Act 1970.[5]

Another case involved a man with Down's Syndrome, whose request to live in a particular residential community had been rejected by the local authority on the basis that it was too expensive. He successfully challenged this decision by means of judicial review. *Disability Now*, the leading disability newspaper, commented: 'Mark Hazell's case is likely to be the forerunner of many others seeking judgement on where the duty of councils really lies.'[6]

Symbolic of this development was the full page article, also in *Disability Now*, encouraging disabled people to use the law to campaign for their rights.[7] Such rights consciousness and litigious mindedness bodes well for the capacity of disabled people to use any future anti-discrimination legislation to the full.

Parliamentary campaigns

The seeds of a new legal approach to disability contained in the Chronically Sick and Disabled Persons Act 1970 (CSDPA) fell on barren ground: this Act was followed by the fall of the Labour government, and four years of Conservative rule in which no legislative progress was made for disabled people in the area of civil rights. When the Labour Party was re-elected in 1974, the CSDPA's author, Alf Morris MP, was named Britain's first Minister for the Disabled, helping to raise the status of disability issues.

In 1977 Morris created a committee to assess the impact of the 1970 Act, focusing particularly on access. The Committee reported in 1979 that there was widespread ignorance of the Act and little improvement in access.[8] It proposed the revision of mandatory building codes to improve access.

A further committee – the Committee on Restrictions against Disabled People (CORAD) – was appointed in 1979 to examine the exclusion of disabled people and propose ways to combat it. CORAD reported in 1982, by which time the Conservatives had again replaced the Labour Party in government.[9] The CORAD Report's most significant recommendation was that broad anti-discrimination legislation should be adopted. However, successive Conservative governments since that date have opposed this recommendation. In 1982, shortly after the publication of the CORAD Report, Jack Ashley MP moved the Disablement Prohibition of Unjustifiable Discrimination Bill. Jack (now Lord) Ashley is a veteran campaigner for the rights of disabled people, having himself become deaf in the middle of his parliamentary career. The

Bill was a short Private Members Bill, giving powers to the Equal Opportunities Commission (EOC) to investigate cases of discrimination against disabled people and seek to resolve them by conciliation. The definition of discrimination was to be determined by the EOC. As a Private Members Bill, low on the ballot, it failed even to achieve substantial debating time in the House of Commons.

In the next session the same Bill was reintroduced by Donald Stewart MP. This time, because of Mr Stewart's high position in the Private Members ballot, a more substantial debate on the Bill took place. However, the government's opposition to the Bill doomed it to failure. The government's position was that education rather than legal penalties was required to stop discrimination.

In the next parliamentary session Robert Waring MP introduced a Bill which sought to achieve the same end by amending the CSDPA to establish a Disablement Commission, which would investigate complaints of discrimination. Individuals were to be given the right to take legal action on their own behalf, and the powers of the Commission were to be left to be defined at a later date. Again the government stopped the Bill progressing beyond its Second Reading. In 1984 a further Bill was introduced, this time in the House of Lords by Lord Campbell of Croy. This Bill would have simply established a Disablement Commission to investigate and review discrimination on the basis of disability. Ian Bynoe, the Legal Director of MIND (the national mental health charity) has described the main difficulties with all these attempts at introducing anti-discrimination laws as being that 'important provisions were left to be defined later by regulation, and that the definitions included in the Bill lacked sophistication or were incomplete'.[10]

A further significant landmark in the equal rights campaign was the formation in 1985 of a coordinating committee of disability organisations, Voluntary Organisations for Anti-Discrimination Legislation (VOADL). VOADL has since been coordinating the lobbying activities aimed at achieving anti-discrimination legislation and has made impressive progress.

In 1991 two important contributions to the campaign were published – Colin Barnes' extensive research project exhaustively documented the institutionalised discrimination against disabled people, and a pamphlet from the Institute for Public Policy Research outlining the arguments for anti-discrimination legislation.[11] I have relied on the foundations contained in these two works in writing this book. Ian Bynoe also played a leading role in drafting on behalf of VOADL the recent series of anti-discrimination Bills. These mark further significant progress, since they are much more detailed and sophisticated than previous Bills. As we have seen, they are also heavily influenced by the provisions of the Americans with Disabilities Act 1990.

The Civil Rights (Disabled People) Bill was introduced as a Private Members Bill at the end of 1991. The Bill reached its Second Reading in February 1992, two months before a general election which would clearly be fiercely contested between the ruling Conservative Party and its chief opposition, the Labour Party. In consequence, the Conservatives did not feel able openly to oppose the Bill (itself a tremendous testimony to the strength of the campaign), but instead arranged for Robert Hayward, a Conservative backbencher, to 'talk out' the Bill.[12] In the event the Conservatives won the election, although Hayward lost his seat.

The Bill was reintroduced in the next session, only to be defeated again at its Second Reading. This time Nicholas Scott, the Conservative Minister for Disabled People, openly opposed the Bill. It is significant that the emphasis of his argument turned not on the lack of need for such legislation, as had previously been the case, but on the issues of costs and comprehensiveness. It was argued that comprehensive anti-discrimination legislation would be too expensive, but that a 'sector by sector approach' to 'tackling discrimination' could be considered.[13]

A further sign of the accelerating political momentum behind the campaign was that, rather than dismissing the call for legislation outright, the Minister offered to liaise with the All Party Disablement Group on 'whether, and if so how, legislation could play any part in seeking to reduce or eliminate discrimination against disabled people'.[14] (This cross-party group of MPs, with veteran campaigners such as Lord Ashley and Alf Morris, has acted as an invaluable focus for the parliamentary campaign.)

Although these discussions took place off the public record, a number of disability organisations were contacted by Scott's office in the following months, asking for proposals for improvements to legislation. The emphasis was on piecemeal improvements which could be made without any cost. There have been no visible signs of progress as a result of these approaches. On the contrary, 1993 saw existing provisions threatened by the government's emphasis on deregulation. The building industry, which has close links with the Conservative Party and is currently represented on a deregulation task force, is known to favour the removal of Part M of the Building Regulations. The privatisation of British Rail and the proposed deregulation of taxis threaten to jeopardise progress towards access in precisely those areas where it has begun to have some, albeit slight, impact.

In response to this lack of progress, the Civil Rights (Disabled Persons) Bill was reintroduced in late 1993 as a Private Members Bill by Dr Roger Berry MP (Labour). The campaign backing this Bill, the third in successive years, was to prove the most successful to date, producing an enormous breakthrough in political support and media attention.

The distribution of 250,000 postcards in support of the Bill, and a lobby of Parliament by over 2,000 disabled people, secured a Second Reading vote of 231 for and none against. The government was forced into a defensive position by which they sought to avoid open opposition to the Bill, and the Bill emerged from its Committee stage without a single opposing amendment being put forward. (Indeed the Bill was strengthened by a number of amendments, most notably extending the employment provisions to all employers.)

Internal sources suggest that the Cabinet was divided in its response to the Bill, with the chief opposition coming from the Departments of Environment and Trade and Industry, and the Prime Minister remaining undecided until a very late stage. The blow finally came at Report stage. The government, still reluctant to be seen to oppose this popular measure, used a handful of backbench Tory MPs to place over 80 wrecking amendments. This ensured that the Bill ran out of the time necessary to complete its parliamentary stages, but led to heightened criticism accusing the government of hypocrisy and duplicity. Indeed, the accompanying press furore produced the highest profile yet for the campaign; the Bill became headline news and the media attention lasted for weeks.

The Minister for Disabled People was also forced to announce a further series of consultations on measures to combat disability discrimination, with a view to possible legislation in employment and the provision of goods and services, a Code of Practice for the insurance industry, the extension of building regulations and the establishment of a new advisory body on disability. Barry Sheerman, the Labour Party spokesperson on disability rights, described these proposals: 'This shabby little effort, this white rabbit which has been picked out of the hat today by the Minister, is not a piece of anti-discrimination legislation but an excuse for not giving the House the right to vote for what disabled people want.'[15]

Employment or comprehensive legislation?

The most significant progress towards anti-discrimination legislation has been made in the employment field. An amendment was moved to the Employment Bill 1989 which would have made discrimination on the basis of disability illegal, but was again defeated by government opposition. In July 1990 the Department of Employment issued a consultative document entitled 'Employment and Training for People with Disabilities'.[16] This was very dismissive of the proposals for anti-discrimination legislation. However, the House of Commons Employment Committee Report took a different view: 'The Government should explore urgently the possibility of equal opportunities legislation for the employment of people with disabilities and report to Parliament on its potential effects and campaign.'[17]

In 1992, the Law Society's Employment Law Committee recommended the introduction of a law protecting disabled people against discrimination in the employment field.[18] It argued that existing laws had failed and voluntary measures were inadequate and unreliable. Perhaps most usefully, the report specifically countered the government's argument that such legislation would not be feasible: 'The substantive law contained in the ADA is well explained and defined and the concepts in the legislation could easily transfer into UK law.'[19]

At the time of the debate on the Second Reading of the Civil Rights Bill 1992, speculation was rife that legislation covering solely the employment area might be offered as a sop. Indeed, Nicholas Scott hinted at this during the debate itself. The 1994 proposals for consultation point in the same direction.

Perhaps the most surprising breakthrough came in December 1993 when the Employers Forum on Disability announced that it had surveyed its members, including some of Britain's largest employers, and that they supported the introduction of anti-discrimination in the employment area.[20] (Comprehensive legislation was said to be an unrealistic goal in the current political climate.) The Institute of Directors also announced its support for this principle.[21]

Both VOADL and the All Party Disablement Group have indicated their opposition to a law confined solely to the employment sphere. It is clear that such a law could only have a limited and distorted impact on the discrimination faced by disabled people. Without access to integrated education at all levels, to accessible transport, homes and the assistance required for independent living in the community, disabled people will continue to be barred from even entering the labour market, never mind securing equality of opportunity within it. From a purely tactical point of view it might be argued that securing the anti-discrimination legislation (ADL) principle in one area might make it easier to expand into others. However, it is more likely that it would be used to fragment and diffuse the campaign. Furthermore, since ADL in other areas is likely to have greater resource implications, the government is likely to prove very resistant to expanding the scope. Perhaps most crucially, limiting ADL for disabled people to the employment sphere would perpetuate our status as second-class citizens, unworthy of the same level of protection as is afforded to women and ethnic minorities.

The campaign has succeeded in attracting an oustanding array of allies, as well as growing media support. Both the Liberal Democrats and the Labour Party support the principle, as does the Trades Union Congress. The *New Statesman*, Britain's leading left-wing political journal, observed in 1993 that: 'it is becoming increasingly clear that disabled people have a political voice and that their votes are important.'[22] The most surprising ally of the campaign is perhaps also the most significant one. The *Sun*, Britain's largest circulation popular newspaper, fiercely Conservative in its politics, carried an editorial backing the 1992 Bill and has given the campaign strong support ever since.[23]

Support from such a quarter is eloquent testimony to the capacity of legislation in this area to reach out beyond the normal supporters of equal rights legislation and draw support from the political right. The American example points to the potential for and the importance of framing argument in such a way as to achieve this goal. Before looking at this vital question, I will briefly consider what support campaigners might hope to draw from the European Community.

Europe

We have already seen the impact which EC legislation and court rulings have had on expanding the reach of British sex equality laws. Given this history, and the negative attitudes of successive Conservative governments, it is not surprising that many in the disability movement are looking to Europe for progress on disability rights. It would be a mistake, however, to see the European route as any kind of a short cut.

To an extent the scope for progress via the European Community depends on the overall development of that entity, and in particular the degree of emphasis which will be placed on the social dimension. From its inception as the European Economic Community its primary emphasis has been on facilitating economic development, and this remains the case. Despite the publicity accorded to the Social Chapter of the Maastricht Treaty, the heart of that document was the provisions for monetary union and agreement by the member states to comply with stringent monetarist targets in order to achieve that union. The future of the European project appears unclear at the present time, but if monetary union is achieved, its impact on reduced welfare spending and economic dislocation is likely to be more significant than any progress which may be made through extending the EC's social agenda.

The social dimension

The EC has to date failed to pass a single binding law or Directive concerning disabled people. In part this can be explained by its limited legal powers to make social policy. Whilst the treaties from which the EC derives its powers allow economic decisions to be made on the basis of majority voting in the Council of Ministers (the chief decision-making body of the EC), matters of social policy have had to be made on the basis of unanimity. The issue of women's equality has been exceptional, because the Treaty of Rome included an explicit statement that this was a goal of the EC. (In contrast there is no such explicit statement banning racial discrimination, and hence no progress has been made through the EC on this issue.) In addition, the social provisions of the treaties refer only to improving the living conditions of workers, making no reference to non-workers, including of course many disabled people.

This is why the launch of the Social Chapter in 1989 appeared such a significant development. The chapter set out a number of social goals for the EC, including for the first time a mention of 'non-workers'. It is not, however, legally binding, nor does it extend the EC's powers in the social field. It is fundamentally a statement of good intention. Even so, Britain (alone of the member states) refused to endorse it.

The Social Chapter does specifically mention disabled people. It states that: 'All disabled persons whatever the origin and nature of their disablement, must be entitled to additional concrete measures aimed at improving their social and professional integration.'[24] However, the Social Action Programme, drawn up by the Commission as an outline plan for progressing the aims contained in the Chapter, contained only one proposal out of 50 which specifically addressed the needs of disabled people. This took the form of a draft Directive on the transport to work for workers with reduced mobility. Although described in this narrow way, it would have required progress to be made in creating accessible public transport systems. It was focused on the safety of disabled workers, in order that it could claim to implement health and safety objectives contained within the Single European Treaty, which allows majority voting. However, the British government objected that this was not a sound legal basis, and that in any event a broader approach covering the requirements of all disabled people, not merely workers, was appropriate. The result, however, has been effectively to block progress in this area.

The Maastricht Treaty has strengthened the ability of the EC to legislate in the social sphere, at least for those member states which signed the Social Protocol. Once again, Britain was the only state not to do so.

This annexe allows social policy decisions to be made on the basis of majority voting. Article 2 of the Agreement on Social Policy (the 'social protocol' of the Treaty on European Union) commits the EC to supporting and complementing the activities of the member states in the integration of persons excluded from the labour market. Undoubtedly disabled people would fall within this category, which at least provides a potential inroad for future positive measures. However, it is not clear as yet how the anomalous situation with regard to Britain will be resolved. In theory, Britain will not be bound by any measures passed under the Social Protocol. Nevertheless, in practice, it seems likely that the Commission will continue to seek the agreement of all member states to its social proposals, and only when it has failed to secure this will it consider passing measures under the Social Protocol.

Disability initiatives

The chief focus of EC policy on disability has been through funding programmes, aimed at disadvantaged groups and regions. Probably the nearest that the EC has come to recognising discrimination as a central problem for disabled people is in the employment field. A Recommendation was issued in 1986,[25] encouraging member states to promote equal opportunities, eliminate 'negative discrimination', ensure that disabled people are able to go before 'competent authorities' to establish their rights and receive the necessary assistance to do so, and take positive action in the form of the adoption of quotas, the dissemination of a Code of Good Practice and subsequent monitoring of it.

However, Recommendations are non-binding statements of guidance, and a 1988 Report into the implementation of this Recommendation by the Commission concluded that little progress had been achieved.[26] A year later the Council of Ministers issued its conclusions on the employment of disabled people.[27] It noted the persistence of substantial disadvantage to disabled people in the labour market, and that whilst general measures to stimulate economic growth were undoubtedly necessary to improve the situation they alone would not prove sufficient. It emphasised the need for measures to improve equal opportunities, and considered the prime aim of such measures would be to 'guarantee that no citizen of the Community suffers discrimination with regard to access to vocational training and employment'.[28] The Council invited the Commission to submit proposals to ensure 'better coordination and greater consistency between the measures introduced by the Member States'.[29] The Commission, however, has failed to follow up this clear invitation to propose more binding measures. It would appear that this stems from the low priority afforded to disability issues.

A particular barrier to the passage of EC measures directed at combating discrimination is the persistence of the view that disability is primarily a welfare issue rather than one to be approached from an equal rights perspective. This is reflected in the predominance of quotas as the dominant response to the problems of disabled workers.

Lunt and Thornton, in their recent review of international employment policies for disabled people, contrast the approach of European countries with those of the US, Canada and Australia.[30] The non-European countries have all adopted comprehensive anti-discrimination legislation. In Australia, the Disability Discrimination Act 1992 supplements the anti-discrimination legislation which already exists in most states and territories; in Canada, disability discrimination is banned under the Canadian Human Rights Act 1977, as specifically amended in 1985. The Employment Equity Act and Federal Contractors Programme both encourage positive action for disabled people, amongst other disadvantaged groups. New Zealand has also recently introduced anti-discrimination laws for disabled people.

In contrast, 'the majority of EC countries have an approach to employment promotion which involves legal requirements guided historically by principles of compulsion and exemplified by quota systems and reserved employment.'[31]

It is doubtless significant that calls for comprehensive anti-discrimination legislation are strongest in Britain out of all the EC countries. The closer links between Britain and the English speaking ex-colonies, together with a greater degree of shared political assumptions, are probably responsible for this situation. It may well prove that Britain becomes the beach-head for importing this civil rights approach to disability into the EC in general.

However, to succeed in passing anti-discrimination measures through the institutions of the EC will require disabled people to organise in each of the member states in support of such measures. At present, the level of self-organisation of disabled people varies greatly between the differing countries. A promising new development is the increasing activity of the international organisation of disabled people (Disabled People's International) at the European level. Thus 1993 saw the first European conference of disabled people and the first European day of action of disabled people. Both of these events demanded that the Commission should pass Directives implementing civil rights for disabled people.

The establishment by the Commission of a Disability Forum, including representatives of disabled people from all twelve nation states, should also assist in ensuring that disability issues achieve more prominence and that they are approached from a rights perspective.

A final important development is the recognition of the European trade union movement that disability is a civil rights issue. Also in 1993, the first European Trades Union Congress (ETUC) conference on disability adopted a recommendation to work towards anti-discrimination legislation, and to work with the organisations of disabled people in order to achieve this.

The prospects for a disability discrimination law

It is becoming increasingly apparent that the opposition of the government to anti-discrimination legislation for disabled people is not one of principle, but one based solely on cost considerations. Whilst it is equally apparent that the campaign for such a law is gaining sufficient momentum to make the political costs of such opposition high, this in itself may not be sufficient to secure victory.

The American example can once again provide a lesson from which the British disability movement could profitably learn. The American movement combined radical activists, who succeeded in raising public and political awareness of the issue, with sophisticated lobbying which succeeded in recasting the issue in ways calculated to appeal to a Republican administration.

In order to understand fully the forces behind the development of anti-discrimination legislation for disabled people it is helpful to return to basics – the analysis of disability contained in Chapter 1. Since the structural exclusion of disabled people from society is a dynamic process, reflecting technological and social as well as political developments, it follows that shifts in these spheres are likely to produce alterations in the positions of people with disabilities. This is not to say that these shifts automatically led to the development of anti-discrimination legislation, but rather that they created the potential for change which an increasingly powerful disability movement was able to utilise to tremendous effect.

At the most basic level, the changing demographics of disability have an impact; the ageing population, in particular, has expanded the numbers of disabled people. In the context of the politicisation of disability this has translated into the lobbying power described above. It also has important economic and social effects.

The opposition of business groups to the Americans with Disabilities Act was surprisingly muted. A leading newspaper attributed this, in part, to their increasing appreciation of disabled people as a 'new source of labor and customers'.[32] Evan Kemp, the Republican head of the Equal Employment Opportunities Commission, appealed to the business community, traditional Republican supporters, in exactly these terms:

> There are good dollar and cents reasons why businesses should be interested in disabled persons. First, disabled people purchase goods and services just like other consumers ... A smart business person would make sure that his or her business was accessible to and useable by disabled people ... 36 million Americans ... can be a profitable market for you.[33]

The other side of the picture presented by the proponents of the Bill was the forthcoming labour shortage. Bowe estimated that the economy was expected to add 21 million new jobs before the end of the century, but that during the same period the working-age population was expected to grow by just 1–2 per cent, more slowly than at any time since the 1930s.[34] This projected expansion coincides with shifts in employment patterns and with technological improvements which open up new areas of work for many disabled people. The number of jobs in the agricultural and heavy industrial sectors has declined sharply whilst white collar jobs, particularly in the service sector, have risen steeply. With adequate training, disabled people would be well suited to such jobs. Furthermore, new computerised technology has opened up these jobs to disabled people. New machines include scanners that can read documents at eight pages per minute and automatically enter text into a word processor, speech synthesizers that speak aloud words on the screens of computers, telecommunications devices for deaf people that allow them to use the telephone, and computers which permit people to work from home.

These were the arguments used to sell the measure to the business sector. Perhaps the labour force arguments seem flawed at a time of recession, but nevertheless both employers and the state will have to recognise the consequences of the growing proportion of older and disabled people within the workforce and revise their policies accordingly. In Britain the Office of Population Censuses and Surveys (OPCS) calculated that 6 per cent of the working population of Britain is disabled,[35] whilst the Labour Force Survey, using a wider definition, estimates that 14 per cent of the economically active population have a health problem or disability which limits the type of work they can do.[36]

The disability lobby won the federal government's backing at least in part through an appeal to its self-interest in cutting the budget deficit. The 1980s had seen considerable government concern about the rapid escalation of welfare programmes for disabled people. Evan Kemp emphasised this point: 'We can no longer afford to spend $122 billion each year on disability programs, when the vast majority of these programs are designed to keep people from working, to segregate them rather than to rehabilitate and employ them'.[37] Frank Bowe, another veteran campaigner, similarly argues:

> No one has ever said that making America accessible could cost as much as does our inaccessibility now. My best estimate is that lack of access now costs America more than $100 billion each and every year with the costs rising to as much as $200 billion a year within the next decade.[38]

He compares the figures, representing 20 per cent of all social welfare expenditures, with estimates of the costs of barrier removal – $20 billion for ten years. Rather than spending funds on programmes of 'dependence and maintenance', Bowe suggests that the government should use some of that money for independence and self-sufficiency. Such a message could not fail to strike a chord with the Republican Party.

The success of the US disability rights movement lay in their persuading key politicians to look at disability through a fundamentally different perspective, in which extending the rights of disabled people could be seen as promoting key policy goals such as labour market efficiency and curbing the growth of 'welfare dependency'. It achieved this strategic reframing of the debate both through its lobbying power and through political mobilisation in a broader sense.

There are signs that the British disability movement recognises the power of utilising the rhetoric of the right. Barnes, for instance, writes about:

> Enabling disabled people to free themselves from unnecessary and costly bureaucratic regulations; to earn a living rather than live off the state; to achieve a degree of personal autonomy comparable to that of non-disabled peers; and to expand their role as consumers.[39]

Scott emphasises the business case for extending civil rights to disabled people:

> The economy suffers by effectively excluding a market of 6.5 million disabled people through inaccessible products, shops, restaurants, pubs, cinemas, sports and recreation facilities and transport. In an article in *The Times* the estimated loss to tourism alone was put at £22.4 billion a year. In July 1993, *Marketing Weekly* identified disabled people as an enormous untapped market ... disabled people's spending power is estimated at approximately £33 billion.[40]

As in America, concerns over the expansion of the welfare state in Britain could provide the crucial impetus for the government to accept that a fundamental redefinition of the concept of disability is required. This would not be surprising, given the welfare state's historical contribution to the construction of a disabled identity, described in Chapter 1.

In Britain the need to restructure the welfare state is now at the heart of the political agenda of both leading parties. Given the centrality of disabled people as clients of the welfare state (and once again the comparison with women is interesting), it is not surprising to find that disabled people have been lined up as one of the key targets for cuts in benefits and services.

If disabled people are to avoid becoming the victims of such restructuring, it is essential that we act now to shift the entire perspective in which the discussion is currently being held, from one in which disabled persons are seen as a burden on society to one in which we are seen as an untapped asset. The aim must be to preserve the beneficial assets of a collectivist approach (which has been dominant in Britain), marrying this with a rights approach (which has been dominant in America). If this could be achieved it would be a tremendously powerful weapon for combating the historical under-privilege of disabled people, backing rights with resources and infusing the welfare system with a respect for their rights and autonomy.

One of the themes running through this book has been the juxta-position of the American rights-based approach to disability with the needs-based approach which dominates the British welfare system. The value of the adoption of an equal rights framework for disability policy has been strongly urged. However, this should not be taken to suggest that the solution lies entirely within the American approach, nor that the British system does not have features which could make vital con-tributions to the American model. At various points in the text the importance of a collective approach to social responsibility, which char-acterises the British welfare system, has been stressed as an essential supplement to the equal rights approach.

An acceptance of social responsibility counters the dangers of indi-vidualism inherent in the rights discourse, providing the justification for measures such as affirmative action which are necessary to achieve real progress towards unravelling the consequences of disadvantage. Similarly the provision of state resources for enforcing the law, through the legal aid system, through sufficiently resourced advocacy groups of disabled people and through adequately funded strategic enforce-ment agencies, is the precondition for achieving change.

Having emphasised the important role which political lobbyists must play in reformulating the terms of the debate, I want to return to the importance of a militant disability movement. The American disability lobby was able to make its powerful intervention because it was seen to be at the front of an increasingly cohesive and articulate disability movement. This was itself a product of the dynamic deve-lopment of a rights discourse contained in the Rehabilitation Act, and the struggle to enforce those rights. Its role is not merely to provide the foot-soldiers for the campaign. For an anti-discrimination law to have any real capacity to achieve its goals it must be the product and instrument of a powerful collective movement. As one gay disability activist has observed: 'If you don't have the grass roots activity, then anything you win at legislative level can easily be lost.'[41]

The right to equal treatment, even with the added understanding that such treatment must value and take into account differences and diversities,[42] is not the solution to all the social problems faced by disabled people. Just as feminists have argued that the assertion of equal rights needs to be supplemented by 'positive rights', so a strong framework of collective provision of housing, transport, health services and education is essential for those whose needs cannot be met within the wage-labour system. Otherwise disabled people who cannot par-ticipate in the labour market or whose needs involve additional expenditure will continue to face the choice of being singled out for 'special treatment', with the inevitable rationing of this through pro-fessional control, or of having an equal portion of an inadequate pie.

This is not an argument against the equal rights approach. That has succeeded in producing an invaluable shift in the ideology of 'disability', moving the law in this area away from its previous emphasis on curing and rehabilitating 'defective' individuals to one on curing society, by removing the barriers to participation by disabled people. Rather, this argument is intended as a warning of the need to go beyond the American model and to link up with other 'disadvantaged' groups to defend and extend the welfare state within this new framework. The most important attribute of the rights ethos is its ability to stimulate the collective self-organisation of disabled people, upon which ultimately the potential for such progress depends.

Notes

Introduction
1. Union of the Physically Impaired against Segregation (UPIAS), *Fundamental Principles of Disability* (London: UPIAS, 1970) p. 2.
2. R. Burgdorf and C. Bell, *Accommodating the Spectrum of Abilities* (Washington, DC: US Commission for Civil Rights, 1983) p. 23.
3. Ann Scales, 'The Emergence of Feminist Jurisprudence', *Yale Law Review* 85 (1986) p. 1378.

Chapter 1: Disability and discrimination
1. The definition put forward by Disabled People's International, as quoted in Colin Barnes, *Disabled People in Britain and Discrimination: A Case for Anti-Discrimination Legislation* (London: Hurst, 1991) p. 2.
2. See Conference of Indian Organizations, *Double Bind: To be Disabled and Asian* (London: London Conference of Indian Organizations, 1987); K. Hearn, 'Disabled Lesbians are Here to Stay', in T. Kaufman and P. Lincoln (eds), *High Risk Lives* (Bridport: Prism Press, 1991); S. Lonsdale, *Women and Disability* (London: Macmillan, 1990); J. Morris, *Able Lives: Women's Experience of Paralysis* (London: Women's Press, 1989); Royal Association in Aid of Deaf People (RAD), *A Change in Approach: A Report on the Experiences of Deaf People from Black and Ethnic Minorities* (London: RAD, 1991); M. Saxton and Florence Howe (eds), *With Wings* (London: Virago, 1988).
3. Committee on Restrictions against Disabled People, *Report by the Committee on Restrictions against Disabled People* (Southampton: HMSO, 1982) p. 7.
4. Colin Barnes, *Disabling Imagery and the Media: An Exploration of the Principles for Media Representations of Disabled People* (Clay Cross: British Council of Organisations of Disabled People [BCODP] 1992); A. Gartner and T. Joe, *Images of the Disabled: Disabling Images* (New York: Praeger, 1987); D. Kent, 'In Search of a Heroine: Images of Women with Disabilities in Fiction and Drama', in A. Asch and M. Fine (eds), *Women with Disabilities: Essays in Psychology, Culture and Politics* (Philadelphia: Temple University Press, 1988).

5. Jenny Morris, *Pride against Prejudice: Transforming Attitudes to Disability* (London: Women's Press, 1991).

6. Ibid. pp. 19–21.

7. Ibid. p. 21.

8. Ibid. p. 29.

9. Ibid.

10. H. Hahn, *Issues of Equality: European Perceptions of Employment Policy and Disabled Persons* (New York: World Rehabilitation Fund, 1984) p. 24.

11. Disabled Persons Transport Advisory Committee, *Public Transport and the Missing Six Millions: What Can be Learned?* (London: DPTAC, 1989).

12. 'No Go', *Which?* June 1990, pp. 347–50.

13. Disabled Persons Transport Advisory Committee, *Making Buses More Suitable for Elderly and Ambulant Disabled People* (London: DPTAC, 1988).

14. J. Wagstaff, 'Getting Around London', *Contact* 65 (1990) pp. 35–6.

15. 'No Go', *Which?*

16. A. Rowe (ed.), *Lifetime Homes: Flexible Housing for Successive Generations* (London: Helen Hamlyn Foundation, 1990).

17. Linda Laurie, *Conference Report: Building Our Lives, Housing, Independent Living and Disabled People* (London: Shelter, 1991) p. 9.

18. Access Committee for England, *Building Homes for Successive Generations* (London: Access Committee for England, 1992).

19. Employment Department, *Labour Force Survey*, March 1993.

20. J. Martin, A. White and H. Meltzer, *Disabled Adults: Services, Transport and Employment* (London: Office of Population Censuses and Surveys, 1989).

21. Ibid.

22. P. Prescott Clarke, *Employment and Handicap* (London: Social and Community Planning Research, 1990) p. 34.

23. Ibid.

24. M. Kettle, *Survey of the Association of Disabled Professionals* (Surrey: Association of Disabled Professionals, 1975).

25. M. Kettle, *Disabled People and their Employment: A Review of Research into the Performance of Disabled People at Work* (Surrey: Association of Disabled Professionals, 1979).

26. United States Department of Labor, *The Performance of Physically Impaired Workers in Manufacturing Industries* (Washington, DC: US Department of Labor, 1948).

27. S. Honey, N. Meager and M. Williams, *Employers' Attitudes towards People with Disabilities* (Brighton: Institute of Manpower Studies, University of Sussex, 1993).

28. Ibid. p. 37.

29. Fifty-two per cent of employers in the survey thought that a lack of suitable premises was the chief problem faced in employing disabled people. See also J. Morrel, *The Employment of People with Disabilities: Research into the Policies and Practices of Employers* (Sheffield: Employment Department, 1990).

30. Ibid.

31. Law Society Solicitors with Disabilities Group, 'Survey', *Educare*, November 1992.

32. 'CSP Pledge on Equality Issues', *Therapy Weekly*, 20 November 1992.

33. Morrel, *Employment of People with Disabilities*.

34. Law Society Solicitors with Disabilities Group, 'Survey'.

35. According to Prescott Clarke, *Employment and Handicap*, 29 per cent of those out of work wanted part-time work.

36. Ibid.

37. Ibid.

38. J. Martin, H. Meltzer and D. Elliott, *The Prevalence of Disability Amongst Adults* (London: Office of Population Censuses and Surveys [OPCS], 1988).

39. H. Brown and H. Smith, 'Whose Life is it Anyway? Community Care Policy', *Disability, Handicap and Society* 4 (1989) p. 110.

40. L. Doyal with Imogen Pennell, *The Political Economy of Health* (London: Pluto Press, 1979) p. 34.

41. Michel Foucault, *Madness and Civilisation: A History of Insanity in the Age of Reason* (London: Tavistock, 1967); Thomas Szaz, *The Myth of Mental Illness* (New York: Harper & Row, 1961); Peter Sedgwick, *Psycho Politics* (London: Pluto Press, 1982).

42. Employment Committee, House of Commons, First Report: *Disability and Employment* (House of Commons Paper 35, 1990) p. vi.

43. V. Finklestein, *Attitudes and Disabled People: Issues for Discussion* (New York: World Rehabilitation Fund, 1980).

44. M. Oliver, *The Politics of Disablement* (Basingstoke: Macmillan, 1990).

45. G. Fulcher, *Disabling Policies? A Comparative Approach to Education Policy and Disability* (London: Falmer, 1989).

46. P. Squibb, 'A Theoretical Structuralist Approach to Special Education', in L. Barton and S. Tomlinson (eds), *Special Education: Policy, Practices and Social Issues* (London: Harper & Row, 1981) p. 43.

47. M. Oliver, 'The Social and Political Context of Educational Policy: The Case of Special Needs', in Len Barton (ed.), *The Politics of Special Educational Needs* (London: Falmer, 1988) p. 18.

48. Barton and Tomlinson (eds), *Special Education: Policy, Practices and Social Issues* p. 19.

49. Income Support (General) Regulations 1987.

50. *Foster* v. *Chief Adjudication Officer*, House of Lords, *Guardian*, 29 January 1993.
51. Robert Scott, *The Making of Blind Men: A Study of Adult Socialization* (New York: Russell Sage Foundation, 1969).
52. H. Liggett, 'Stars are Not Born: An Interactive Approach to the Politics of Disability', *Disability, Handicap and Society* 3(3) (1988) p. 271, quoting I. Howards, H. Brahm and S. Naagi, *Disability from Social Program to Federal Program* (New York: Praeger, 1980).
53. D. Stone, *The Disabled State* (Basingstoke: Macmillan, 1984) p. 26.
54. An excellent analysis of anthropological accounts of disability is in Oliver, *The Politics of Disablement*. See also J. Hanks and L. Hanks, 'The Physically Handicapped in Certain Non-Occidental Societies', in W. Philips and J. Rosenberg (eds), *Social Scientists and the Physically Handicapped* (London: Arno Press, 1980); Gartner and Joe, *Images of the Disabled*; J. Ryan and F. Thomas, *The Politics of Mental Handicap* (Harmondsworth: Penguin, 1980); R. Edgerton, *Deviance: A Cross-Cultural Perspective* (London: Benjamin, 1976); B. Farber, *Mental Handicap: Its Social Context and Social Consequences* (Boston: Houghton Mifflin, 1986).
55. Finklestein, *Attitudes and Disabled People*.
56. Ryan and Thomas, *The Politics of Mental Handicap* p. 101.
57. M. Foucault, *Power/Knowledge: Selected Interviews and Other Writings 1972–77* (Brighton: Wheatsheaf, 1980) p. 172.
58. Oliver, *The Politics of Disablement* p. 46.
59. Doyal, *Political Economy of Health* pp. 34–5.
60. Stone, *The Disabled State* p. 12.
61. Brown and Smith, 'Whose Life is it Anyway?', p. 109.
62. M. Foucault, *Archeology of Knowledge* (New York: Pantheon, 1972).
63. Ian Gough, *The Political Economy of the Welfare State* (London: Macmillan, 1981); Elizabeth Wilson, *Only Halfway to Paradise* (London: Tavistock, 1980).
64. D. Rothman, *The Discovery of the Asylum* (Boston, Mass.: Little, Brown, 1971).
65. Stone, *The Disabled State* p. 39.
66. See Stone, *The Disabled State* and M.A. Crowther, *The Workhouse System 1834–1929: The History of an English Institution* (London: Methuen, 1983).
67. J. Gibbons, 'Residential Care for Mentally Ill Adults', in I. Sinclair (ed.), *Residential Care: The Research Reviewed*, literature surveys commissioned by the Independent Review of Residential Care (London: National Institute for Social Work/HMSO, 1988) p. 160.
68. Sinclair (ed.), *Residential Care: The Research Reviewed* p. 128.
69. F. Harrison, *The Young Disabled Adult: The Use of Residential Homes and Hospital Units for the Age Group 16–64: A Report for the Royal College of Physicians* (London: Royal College of Physicians, 1986).

70. F. Bowe, *Handicapping America* (New York: Harper & Row, 1978) p. 170.
71. Doyal, *Political Economy of Health* p. 147.
72. Foucault, *Madness and Civilisation*; I. Illich, *Medical Nemesis: The Expropriation of Health* (London: Calder & Boyars, 1975).
73. Oliver, *The Politics of Disablement* p. 48.
74. Mike Oliver, 'Cock-up or Conspiracy?', *Therapy Weekly*, 11 March 1993.
75. R. Scotch, *From Goodwill to Civil Rights: Transforming Federal Disability Policy* (Philadelphia: Temple University Press, 1984) p. 24.
76. Scotch, *From Goodwill to Civil Rights* p. 6.
77. Ibid.
78. Katzman, *Institutional Disability: The Saga of Transportation Policy for the Disabled* (Washington, DC: Brookings Institute, 1986) p. 110.
79. Scotch, *From Goodwill to Civil Rights*; and S. Percy, *Disability, Civil Rights and Public Policy: The Politics of Implementation* (Montgomery: University of Alabama Press,1989).
80. Peter Libassi, quoted in Scotch, *From Goodwill to Civil Rights* p. 114.
81. Katzman, *Institutional Disability* p. 111.
82. Scotch, *From Goodwill to Civil Rights* p. 150.

Chapter 2: Law's power over inequality

1. Alan Thomson, 'Foreword: Critical Approaches to Law: Who Needs Legal Theory?', in I. Grigg-Spall and P. Ireland (eds), *The Critical Lawyers Handbook* (London: Pluto Press, 1992) p. 4.
2. P. Fitzpatrick, 'Racism and the Innocence of Law', in P. Fitzpatrick and A. Hunt (eds), *Critical Legal Studies* (Oxford: Blackwell, 1987) p. 120.
3. Ibid.
4. C. Gilligan, *In a Different Voice* (London: Harvard University Press, 1982).
5. C. Smart, *Feminism and the Power of Law* (London: Routledge, 1989) p. 86.
6. R. Cotterell, *The Sociology of Law: An Introduction*, 2nd edn. (London: Butterworths, 1992) p. 64.
7. L. Lustgarten and J. Edwards, 'Racial Equality and the Limits of the Law', in P. Braham, A. Rattansi and R. Skellington (eds), *Racism and Anti-Racism: Inequalities, Opportunities and Policies* (London: Sage, 1992) p. 277.
8. Smart, *Feminism and the Power of Law* p. 88.
9. E. Pashunakis, *Law and Marxism: A General Theory* (London: Ink Links, 1987).
10. Cotterell, *Sociology of Law* p. 119.
11. Race Relations Act 1976, Section 1.1.a.

12. J. Conaghan and W. Mansell, 'Tort Law', in Grigg-Spall and Ireland (eds), *Critical Lawyers Handbook* p. 87.
13. C. Lawrence, 'The Id, Ego and Equal Protection: Reckoning with Unconscious Racism', *Stanford Law Review* 39 (1987) p. 324.
14. A. Scales, 'The Emergence of Feminist Jurisprudence', *Yale Law Journal* 95 (1986) p. 1378.
15. L. Dickens, *Whose Flexibility? Discrimination and Equality Issues in Atypical Work* (London: Institute of Employment Rights, 1992) p. 5.
16. Lustgarten and Edwards, 'Racial Inequality and the Limits of Law' p. 273.
17. V. Fuchs, *Women's Quest for Equality* (Cambridge, Mass.: Harvard University Press, 1980).
18. D. Treiman and H. Hartman, *Women, Work and Wages* (Washington, DC: National Academy Press, 1981).
19. TUC, *Women in the Labour Market* (London: TUC, 1983).
20. Equal Opportunities Commission (EOC), *Women and Men in Britain: A Statistical Profile* (Manchester: EOC, 1986).
21. Dickens, *Whose Flexibility?* p. 5.
22. A. Spencer and D. Podmore, *In a Man's World: Essays on Women in Male Dominated Professions* (London: Tavistock, 1987); Anne Witz, *Professions and Patriarchy* (London: Routledge, 1992); R. Compton and K. Sanderson, *Gendered Jobs and Social Change* (London: Unwin Hyman, 1990).
23. *Singh* v. *The Chief Constable of the Nottingham Constabulary CID*, referred to in Commission for Racial Equality (CRE), *Second Review of the Race Relations Act 1976: A Consultative Paper* (London: CRE, 1991).
24. J. Gardner, *No Offence?* (London: Industrial Society, 1993).
25. Dickens, *Whose Flexibility?*
26. Smart, *Feminism and the Power of Law*.
27. An American case considered precisely this point, *Boyd* v. *Ozark Airlines* 568 F. 2d 50, 8th Cir. (1977).
28. J. Gregory, *Sex, Race and the Law: Legislating for Equality* (London: Sage, 1987) p. 16.
29. M. Eastwood, 'The Double Standard of Justice: Women's Rights under the Constitution', *Valparaiso University Law Review* 5(2) (1971) p. 509.
30. L. Krieger and P. Cooney, 'The Miller Wohl Controversy: Equal Treatment, Positive Action and the Meaning of Women's Equality', *Golden Gate University Law Review* 13 (513) (1983).
31. Catharine MacKinnon, *Feminism Unmodified: Discourses on Life and Law* (Cambridge, Mass.: Harvard University Press, 1987).

32. N. Taub and W. Williams, 'Will Equality Require more than Assimilation, Accommodation or Separation from the Existing Strucure?', *Rutger Law Review* 37 (1987) p. 832.
33. Martha McCluskey, 'Rethinking Equality and Difference: Disability Discrimination in Public Transport', *Yale Law Journal* 97 (1988).
34. L. Finley, 'Transcending Equality Theory: A Way out of the Maternity and Workplace Debate', *Columbia Law Review* 86 (1986).
35. McCluskey, 'Rethinking Equality and Difference'.
36. *Griggs* v. *Duke Power Co.* 401 US 424 (1971).
37. Ibid.
38. Ibid.
39. Ibid.
40. M. Eichner, 'Getting Women Work which isn't Women's Work: Challenging Biases in the Workplace', *Yale Law Journal* 97 (1988).
41. J. Brodin, 'Cost, Profit and the Equal Opportunity', *Notre Dame Law Review* 62 (1987) argues that this reluctance reflects the continuing dominance of the intent/fault model for discrimination law.
42. Race Relations Act 1976, Section 1(b).
43. Sex Discrimination Act 1975, Section 1(b).
44. Commission for Racial Equality, *Second Review of the Race Relations Act* (London: CRE, 1992) p. 18.
45. Ibid.
46. Ibid. p. 19.
47. E. Meehan, *Women's Rights at Work: Campaigns and Policy in Britain and the United States* (Basingstoke: Macmillan, 1985) p. 180.
48. *United Papermakers and Paperworkers* v. *United States* 397 US 919 (1970); Gregory, *Sex, Race and the Law* p. 49.
49. A. Blumenrosen, 'The Legacy of Griggs: Social Progress and Subjective Judgment', *Chicago–Kent Law Review* 82 (1986).
50. Meehan, *Women's Rights at Work* p. 174.
51. Duncan Kennedy, 'Legal Education as Training for Hierarchy', in Grigg-Spall and Ireland (eds), *Critical Lawyers Handbook* pp. 57–8.
52. Smart, *Feminism and the Power of Law* p. 143.
53. Scotch, *From Goodwill to Civil Rights: Transforming Federal Disability Policy* (Philadelphia: Temple University Press, 1984) pp. 42–3.
54. Smart, *Feminism and the Power of Law*.
55. Patricia Williams, 'Alchemical Notes: Reconstructing Ideals from Deconstructed Rights', *Harvard Civil Rights–Civil Liberties Review* 22 (1987) p. 416.
56. Elizabeth Schneider, 'The Dialectics of Rights and Politics: Perspectives from the Women's Movement', *New York Univ. Law Review* 61 (1986) p. 626.
57. Ibid. p. 590.

58. H. Liggett, 'Stars are Not Born: An Interactive Approach to the Politics of Disability', *Disability, Handicap and Society* 3 (3) (1988) p. 271.

59. J. Weeks, *Sex, Politics and Society: The Regulation of Sexuality since 1800*, 2nd edn. (London: Longman, 1989).

60. Smart, *Feminism and the Power of Law* p. 165.

61. *City of Cleburne* v. *Cleburne Living Center* 473 US 432 (1985).

62. Ibid.

63. R. Burgdorf and C. Bell, *Accommodating the Spectrum of Abilities* (Washington, DC: US Commission for Civil Rights, 1983) p. 23.

64. M. Martin, 'Note: Accommodating the Handicapped: The Meaning of Discrimination under s504 of the Rehabilitation Act', *New York University Law Review* 55 (1980) pp. 881–906.

65. Ian Bynoe, Mike Oliver and Colin Barnes, *Equal Rights for Disabled People – The Case for a New Law* (London: Institute for Public Policy Research, 1991).

66. *Southeastern Community College* v. *Davis* 442 US 397 (1979).

67. M. Rebell, 'Structural Discrimination and the Disabled', *Georgetown Law Journal* 74 (1986) p. 1451.

68. 'Maternity Proposals Will Increase Sex Bias', *Equal Opportunities Review*, no. 52 (November/December 1993) p. 4.

69. Brodin, 'Cost, Profit and the Equal Opportunity'.

70. National Council on Disability, *Towards Independence* (Washington, DC: National Council on Disability, 1986).

71. Lustgarten and Edwards, 'Limits of the Law'.

72. Ibid. p. 272.

73. Finley, 'Transcending Equality Theory' p. 1159.

74. V. Finklestein, *Attitudes and Disabled People: Issues for Discussion* (New York: World Rehabilitation Fund, 1980) p. 15.

75. H. Hahn, *Issues of Equality: European Perceptions of Employment Policy and Disabled Persons* (New York: World Rehabilitation Fund,1984).

76. Richard Scotch, 'Disability Politics and Disability Rights: A Perspective from Great Britain' (unpublished Fellowship Report for the World Rehabilitation Fund, 1986) p. 21.

Chapter 3: The structure of American disability laws

1. Rehabilitation Act 1973, Section 504.

2. *CQ Researcher*, 'The Disabilities Act', 1 (32) 27 December 1991, p. 999.

3. *Alexander, Governor of Tennesse et al.* v. *Choate* 469 US 287 (1985).

4. *Southeastern Community College* v. *Davis* 442 US 397 (1979).

5. Ibid.

6. Ibid.

7. *Alexander* v. *Choate*.

8. Ibid.
9. Ibid.
10. Ibid.
11. *School Board of Nassau County, Florida* v. *Arline* 480 US 273 (1987).
12. Ibid.
13. Ibid.
14. *Smith* v. *Barton* 914 F.2d 1330 (1990).
15. Ibid.
16. *Texas Dept of Community Affairs* v. *Burdine* 450 US 248 (1981).
17. Ibid.
18. Ibid.
19. Amy Gittler, 'Fair Employment and the Handicapped: A Legal Perspective', *De Paul Law Review* 27 (1978) p. 971.
20. Ibid.
21. Ibid.
22. Ibid.
23. E. Yellin, 'The Recent History and Immediate Future of Employment amongst People with Disabilities, in J. West, *Millbank Quarterly* 69 (1991).
24. *Weeks* v. *Southern Bell Telephone & Telegraph Company* 408 F.2. 228 (1971).
25. Ibid.
26. *Gurmakin* v. *Costyanzo* 556 F.2d. 184 (1977).
27. *Drennon* v. *Philadelphia General Hospital* 428 F.Supp. 809 (1977).
28. *Garrity* v. *Galen* 522 F.Supp. 171 (1981).
29. *Doe* v. *New York University* 666 F.2d. 761 (1981).
30. *Boynton Cab Co.* v. *Dept. of Industry, Labor and Human Relations* 96 Wis.2d. 396 (1980).
31. *Costner* v. *US Dept of Transportation* 555 F.Supp. 146 (1982).
32. Ibid.
33. *School Board of Nassau County, Florida* v. *Arline.*
34. R. Burgdorf and C. Bell, *Accommodating the Spectrum of Abilities* (Washington, DC: US Commission for Civil Rights, 1983) p. 34.
35. *Bentivegna* v. *US Dept of Labor* 694 F.2d. 619 (1982).
36. Ibid.
37. *Stutts* v. *Freeman* 694 F.2d. 666 (1983).
38. ADA Section 102(b)(7).
39. *Bentivegna* v. *US Dept of Labor.*
40. Note: 'Employment Discrimination Against the Handicapped: An Essay in Legal Evasiveness', *Harvard Law Review* 97 (1984) p. 1012.
41. *Bentivegna* v. *US Dept of Labor.*
42. *Pushkin* v. *Regents of the University of Colorado* 658 F.2d 1372 (1981).
43. *Poole* v. *South Painfield Board of Education* 490 F.Supp. 948 (1980).
44. Section 103(b).
45. ADA S. 101 (10).

46. M. Johnson, 'The Rehabilitation Act and Disabled Workers', in M. Berkowitz and A. Hill (eds), *Disability in the Labor Market* (New York: Praeger, 1986).
47. *Prewitt* v. *US Postal Service* 662 F.2d. 292 (5th Cir. 1981).
48. *Transworld Airlines* v. *Hardison* 432 US S.Ct 2277 (1977).
49. *Nelson* v. *Thornborough* 567 F.Supp 369 (1983).
50. Ibid.
51. Ibid.
52. *Smith* v. *Administrator of Veteran Affairs* (32 Fair Emp. Practice Cases CD Cal., 1983).
53. *Dexter* v. *Tisch*, 660 F.Supp. 1418 (D-Conn. 1987).
54. Julie Bradfield, 'Undue Hardship: Title 1 ADA', *Fordham Law Review* 1 (1990) p. 119.
55. 'Employment Act for Lawyers', *Wall Street Journal*, 11 September 1989.
56. Sen. Harken (D-Iowa), 135 Cong Rec S 4986 (9 May 1989).
57. Sen. Helms (R-NC) 135 Cong Rec S10773 (7 September 1989).
58. Note: 'Employment Discrimination Against the Handicapped' p. 1012.
59. S. Gerse, 'Mending the Rehabilitation Act of 1973', *University of Illinois Law Review* (1982).
60. M. McCluskey, 'Rethinking Equality and Difference: Disability Discrimination in Public Transport', *Yale Law Journal* 97 (1988).
61. ADA Section 2.6.
62. A. Rasky, 'How the Disabled Sold Congress on a New Bill of Rights', *New York Times*, 17 September 1989.

Chapter 4: The effectiveness of American disability laws

1. R. Cotterell, *The Sociology of Law: An Introduction*, 2nd edn. (London: Butterworths, 1992) p. 64.
2. A. Lester and G. Bindman, *Race and the Law* (Harmondsworth: Penguin, 1972) p. 24.
3. L. Harris and Associates, *Disabled Americans' Self-Perceptions: Bringing Disabled Americans into the Mainstream* (New York: Harris, 1986).
4. P. Hippololitus, *College Bound Freshmen with Disabilities Preparing for Employment: A Statistical Profile* (Washington, DC: President's Committee on the Employment of the Handicapped and the American Council for Education, 1985) p. 2.
5. R. Katzman, *Institutional Disability: The Saga of Transportation Policy for the Disabled* (Washington, DC: Brookings Institute, 1986).
6. *APTA* v. *Lewis* 655 F.2d 1272 (DC Cir. 1981).
7. US Department of Transportation, *Preliminary Cost Analysis: ADA Vehicle Accessibility Requirements* (Washington, DC: DOT, 1990).

8. E. Yellin, 'The Recent History and Immediate Future of Employment amongst People with Disabilities', in J. West, *Millbank Quarterly* 69 (1991).
9. Ibid. p. 135.
10. Ibid. p. 137.
11. Quoted in an interview in *Business Week*, 28 October 1991.
12. B. Tucker, 'Section 504 of the Rehabilitation Act after Ten Years of Enforcement: The Past and the Future', *University of Illinois Law Review* 4 (1989) p. 915.
13. Ibid. p. 848.
14. *Consolidated Rail Corp.* v. *Darrone* 104 S. Ct 1249 (1984).
15. Tucker, 'Ten Years of Enforcement' p. 878.
16. Ibid.
17. G. Pati and J. Adkins, 'Hire the Handicapped – Compliance is Good Business', *Harvard Business Review*, January 1980 p. 14.
18. Quoted in 'The Disabilities Act', *CQ Researcher*, 1(32), 27 December 1991, p. 999.
19. Quoted in Frank Bowe, *Civil Rights Issues for Handicapped Americans* (New York: Harper & Row, 1980).
20. Bowe, *Civil Rights Issues*, p. 32.
21. Ibid. p. 34.
22. Ibid. p. 36.
23. *Paralyzed Veterans of America et al.* v. *William French Smith et al.*, 27 CCH EPD P32 277 (C.D.Ca. 1981).
24. Pati and Adkins, 'Hire the Handicapped', p. 14.
25. Ibid.
26. R. Scotch, *From Goodwill to Civil Rights: Transforming Federal Disability Policy* (Philadelphia: Temple University Press, 1984); S. Percy, *Disability, Civil Rights and Public Policy: The Politics of Implementation* (Montgomery: University of Alabama Press, 1989); Katzman, *Institutional Disability*.
27. *Grove* v. *Bell* 465 US 555 (1984), overturned by the Civil Rights Restoration Act 1986.
28. National Council on Disability, *Towards Independence* (Washington, DC: National Council on Disability, 1986).
29. National Council on Disability, *On the Threshold of Independence* (Washington, DC: National Council on Disability, 1988).
30. *National Review*, 11 June 1990.
31. Speech to Employers' Banquet of the President's Committee on the Employment of the Handicapped, 5 May 1988.
32. Ibid.
33. Harris, *Bringing Disabled Americans into the Mainstream*.
34. The Telecommunications Accessibility Enhancement Act 1988 expanded the existing pilot Federal Relay Service, applying to calls to and within the Federal government, and required a study

to assess the feasibility of extending this to all interstate calls. The Hearing Aid Compatibility Act 1988 required all new telephones to be compatible with hearing aids. Other laws required television captioning, access to emergency services by TDD (typewriter activated telephones) and improved provision of sign interpreters in court proceedings.

35. ADA s. 308 b 1 B.
36. Mary Johnson, 'Enabling Act: Americans with Disabilities Act', *The Nation*, 28 November 1989.
37. The Gallup Organization, *Baseline Study to Determine Businesses' Attitudes, Awareness and Reaction to the Americans with Disabilities Act* (Princeton, NJ: Gallup, 1992).
38. Victoria Scott, *Lessons from America* (London: Royal Association for Disability and Rehabilitation, 1994).
39. US General Accounting Office, *Report to the Subcommittee on Select Education and Civil Rights, Committee on Education and Labor, House of Representatives: Americans with Disabilities Act, Initial Accessibility Good but Important Barriers Remain* (Washington,DC: US General Accounting Office, 1993).
40. Gallup, *Baseline Study*.
41. National Council on Disability, *ADA Watch – Year One: A Report to the President and Congress on Progress in Implementing the Americans with Disabilities Act* (Washington,DC: National Council on Disability, 1993).
42. Ibid. pp. 2 and 31.
43. Ibid. p. 31.
44. Equal Employment Opportunity Commission, 'EEOC Marks First Year of Enforcing the ADA in the Workplace', press release, Washington, DC, 23 July 1993.
45. Scott, *Lessons from America* p. 26.
46. *USA Today*, 22 July 1993.
47. Johnson, 'Enabling Act'.

Chapter 5: Importing anti-discrimination laws

1. K. Holland, *Judicial Activism in Comparative Perspective* (London: Macmillan, 1991).
2. Alexis de Tocqueville, *Democracy in America*, ed. Phillip Bradley (New York: Knopf, 1945) p. 280.
3. C. Harlow and R. Rawlings, *Pressure through Law* (London: Routledge, 1992) p. 110.
4. Known as the Wednesbury rule, from the case *Associated Provincial Picture Houses Ltd* v. *Wednesbury Corporation* 1 KB 223 1948.
5. J. A. G. Griffith, *The Politics of the Judiciary*, 2nd edn. (London: Fontana, 1981) p. 230.

6. A. Lester and G. Bindman, *Race and the Law* (Harmondsworth: Penguin, 1972).

7. Ibid. p. 39.

8. Ibid. p. 25.

9. *De Costa* v. *Paz* 1954 Amb 228.

10. *Commissioner for Local Government Lands and Settlement* v. *Kaderbhai* 1931 AC 652.

11. Lester and Bindman, *Race and the Law* p. 46.

12. *Nagle* v. *Fielden* [1966] 2 QB 633 (CA).

13. Ibid.

14. Ibid.

15. Ibid.

16. Lester and Bindman, *Race and the Law* p. 24.

17. *Brown* v. *Board of Education* 347 US 483 (1954).

18. *Plessey* v. *Ferguson* 163 US 537 (1896).

19. Eric Foner, *A Short History of Reconstruction* (New York: Harper & Row, 1990).

20. *Korematsu* v. *US* 323 US 214 (1944).

21. *Fontiero* v. *Richardson* 411 US 677 (1973); *Craig* v. *Boren* 429 US 190 (1976).

22. *City of Cleburne* v. *Cleburne Living Center* 473 US 432 (1985).

23. *Pennsylania Association for Retarded Children* v. *Commonwealth of Pennsylvania* 343 F.Supp. 280 (1972).

24. *Yongberg* v. *Romeo* 457 US 307 (1982).

25. R. Scotch, *From Goodwill to Civil Rights: Transforming Federal Disability Policy* (Philadelphia: Temple University Press, 1984) p. 153.

26. R. Unger, *Critical Legal Studies Movement* (Cambridge, Mass.: Harvard University Press, 1986).

27. Holland, *Judicial Activism*.

28. R. Scotch, 'Disability Politics and Disability Rights: A Perspective from Great Britain' (unpublished Fellowship Report for World Rehabilitation Fund, 1986) p. 13.

29. E. Meehan, *Women's Rights at Work: Campaigns and Policy in Britain and the United States* (Basingstoke: Macmillan, 1985); R. Dahl, *Dilemmas of Pluralist Democracy: Autonomy and Control* (New Haven, Conn.: Yale University Press, 1982).

30. Harlow and Rawlings, *Pressure through Law* p. 94.

31. Scotch, *From Goodwill to Civil Rights* p. 133.

32. Harlow and Rawlings, *Pressure through Law* p. 6.

33. Ibid.

34. J. Cooper and R. Dhavan, *Public Interest Law* (Oxford: Blackwell, 1986).

35. L. Gostin (ed.), *Civil Liberties in Conflict* (London: Routledge, 1988).

36. J. Cooper, *Key Guide to Information Sources in Public Law* (London: Mansell,1991).
37. Harlow and Rawlings, *Pressure through Law* p. 298.
38. Holland, *Judicial Activism* p. 41.
39. *Gillick* v. *West Norfolk and Wisbech Area Health Authority* 1985 1 All ER 532.
40. A. Lester, *A British Bill of Rights* (London: Institute of Public Policy Research, 1990).
41. Holland, *Judicial Activism* p. 48.
42. Harlow and Rawlings, *Pressure through Law* pp. 296–7.
43. Adam Sage, 'Black Barristers Face Exam Bias', *Independent*, 10 September 1993.
44. G. Bindman, 'Appointing Judges without Discrimination', *New Law Journal*, 13 December 1991.
45. Lord Chancellor's Department, *Judicial Appointments – The Lord Chancellor's Policies and Procedures*, (London: Lord Chancellor's Department, 1990) p. 5.
46. Bindman, 'Appointing Judges' p. 1693.
47. Commission for Racial Equality, *The Race Relations Code of Practice in Employment* (London: CRE, 1984).
48. Committee on Restrictions against Disabled People, *Report by the Committee on the Restrictions against Disabled People* (Southampton: HMSO, 1982)p. 17.

Chapter 6: British race and sex laws – could do better

1. C. Brown and P. Gay, *Racial Discrimination: 17 Years after the Act* (London: Policy Studies Institute, 1986).
2. 'Ethnic Origins and the Labour Market', *Employment Gazette*, March 1990.
3. *Equal Opportunities Review*, 52, November/December 1993.
4. Commission for Racial Equality, *Second Review of the Race Relations Act 1976* (London: CRE, 1991) p. 29.
5. Race Relations Act 1976 s. 57(3); Sex Discrimination Act 1975 s. 66(3).
6. Sex Discrimination Act s. 66(3) and Race Relations Act s. 57(3).
7. *Price* v. *Civil Service Commission* 1978 IRLR 3.
8. *Holmes* v. *The Home Office* 1984 IRLR 299.
9. *Clarke and Powell* v. *Eley Kynoch* 1982 IRLR 483.
10. *Kidd* v. *DRG (UK) Ltd* 1985 IRLR 190.
11. J. Gregory, *Sex, Race and the Law: Legislating for Equality* (London, Sage: 1987), p. 43.
12. P. Fitzpatrick, 'Racism and the Innocence of Law', in P. Fitzpatrick and A. Hunt (eds), *Critical Legal Studies* (Oxford: Blackwell, 1987).
13. *Ojutiku and Another* v. *Manpower Services Commission* 1982 IRLR 418 CA.

14. *Orphanos* v. *Queen Mary's College* 1985 IRLR 349.
15. *Bilka-Kaufhaus GmbH* v. *Weber von Hartz* Case 170/84 (1986) ECR 1607.
16. *Hampson* v. *DES* 1989 IRLR 69.
17. *Perera* v. *Civil Service Commission* 1983 IRLR 166.
18. Commission for Racial Equality, *Second Review of the Race Relations Act* (London: CRE, 1992); Equal Opportunities Commission, *Equal Treatment for Men and Women, Strengthening the Acts: Formal Proposals* (Manchester: EOC, 1988).
19. C. McCrudden, D. Smith and C. Brown, *Racial Justice at Work: Enforcement of the Race Relations Act 1976* (London: Policy Studies Institute, 1991) p. 136.
20. *Noone* v. *NW Thames Regional Health Authority* (no. 2) 1988 IRLR 530 CA.
21. McCrudden et al., *Justice at Work* p. 176.
22. H. Genn and Y. Genn, *The Effectiveness of Representation at Tribunals: Report to the Lord Chancellor* (London: Lord Chancellor's Department, 1989); V. Kumar, *Industrial Tribunal Applicants under the Race Relations Act 1976* (London: CRE, 1986); J. Gregory, *Trial by Ordeal: A Study of People who Lose Equal Pay and Sex Discrimination Cases in the Industrial Tribunals during 1985 and 1986* (London: HMSO, 1989).
23. T. Eisenberg, 'Integration Models and Trial Outcomes in Civil Rights and Prisoner Cases', *Georgetown Law Review* 77 (1989); B. Curran, *The Legal Needs of the Public* (Chicago: American Bar Foundation, 1977).
24. P. Burstein and K. Monaghan, 'Equal Opportunity and the Mobilization of Law', *Law and Society Review,* 20 (1986).
25. Gregory, *Sex, Race and the Law* p. 75.
26. A. Leonard, *Judging Inequality: The Effectiveness of the Tribunal System in Sex Discrimination and Equal Pay Cases* (London: Cobden Trust, 1987).
27. G. Bindman, 'Appointing Judges without Discrimination', *New Law Journal,* 13 December 1991.
28. Ibid.
29. Fitzpatrick, 'Racism and the Innocence of Law' p. 126.
30. *De Souza* v. *The Automobile Association* 1985 IRLR 87, quoted in Gregory, *Sex, Race and the Law* p. 103.
31. M. Drummond, 'Positive Discrimination', *Guardian,* 1 March 1994.
32. *Orphanos* v. *Queen Mary College* 1985 IRLR 349 HL.
33. *Alexander* v. *The Home Office* 1988 IRLR 190 CA.
34. *Bradford Council* v. *Arora* 1991 IRLR 165 CA.
35. Gregory, *Sex, Race and the Law* p. 81.
36. Ibid. p. 278.

37. 'Compensation Awards: Employers Pay More for Race and Sex Bias', *Equal Opportunities Review*, 49, May/June 1993 pp. 11–12.
38. Ibid.
39. *Marshall* v. *SW Hants Health Authority* 1986 IRLR 140 ECJ.
40. *Equal Opportunities Review* November/December 1993.
41. CRE, *Second Review of the Race Relations Act*.
42. E. Meehan, *Women's Rights at Work: Campaigns and Policy in Britain and the United States* (Basingstoke: Macmillan, 1985) p. 178.
43. Race Relations Act Sections 37 and 38; Sex Discrimination Act Sections 47 and 48.
44. Institute of Personnel Management, *Contract Compliance – The UK Experience* (London: Income Data Services, 1987).
45. Local Government Act 1989 Sections 17 and 18.
46. R. Marshall, C. Knapp and R. Glover, *Employment Discrimination: The Impact of Legal and Administrative Remedies* (New York: Praeger, 1978).
47. P. Wallace (ed.), *Equal Employment Opportunity and the AT & T Case* (Cambridge, Mass.: MIT Press, 1976).
48. A. Adams, *Towards Fair Employment and the EEOC: A Study of Compliance Procedures under Title VII of the Civil Rights Act 1965* (Washington, DC: EEOC, 1972); M. Liggett, 'The Efficacy of State Fair Employment Commissions', *Industrial and Labor Relations Research*, 22 (1968–9).
49. G. Chambers and C. Horton, *Promoting Sex Equality: The Role of Industrial Tribunals* (London: Policy Studies Institute, 1990) p. 178.
50. McCrudden et al., *Racial Justice at Work*.
51. Ibid. p. 267.
52. Ibid.
53. Re Prestige 1984 ICR 473.
54. Gregory, *Sex, Race and the Law* p. 115.
55. McCrudden et al., *Racial Justice at Work* p. 111.
56. *Standing Advisory Committee on Human Rights, Religious and Political Discrimination and Equal Opportunity in Northern Ireland* Cm. 237 (London: HMSO, 1987) para. 7.70 (quoted in CRE, *Second Review of the Race Relations Act* p. 37).
57. CRE, *Second Review of the Race Relations Act* p. 40.
58. C. McCrudden, 'The Northern Ireland Fair Employment White Paper: A Critical Assessment, *Industrial Law Journal* 17 (1988).
59. A. Blumenrosen, 'Towards Effective Administration of New Regulatory Statutes, *Administrative Law Review* 2 (1977).
60. Meehan, *Women's Rights at Work*.
61. Ibid. p. 143.
62. Gregory, *Sex, Race and the Law* p. 140.
63. Eric Robinson, quoted in J. Gregory, *Sex, Race and the Law* p. 139.

64. Race Relations Act 1976 Section 20; Sex Discrimination Act 1975 Section 29.
65. McCrudden et al., *Racial Justice at Work* p. 58.
66. Equal Opportunities Commission, *Annual Report 1992: The Equality Challenge* (Manchester: EOC, 1992).
67. Commission for Racial Equality, *Race through the 90s* (London: CRE, 1993) p. 14.
68. Equal Opportunities Commission, *Equal Treatment for Men and Women* p. 19.
69. McCrudden et al., *Racial Justice at Work* p. 106.
70. Race Relations Act Section 71.
71. Equal Opportunities Commission, *Equal Treatment for Men and Women*, p. 15.
72. Commission for Racial Equality, *Race and Council Housing in Hackney: Report of a Formal Investigation* (London: CRE, 1984); Commission for Racial Equality, *Race and Housing in Liverpool*, 2nd edn. (London: CRE, 1986); Commission for Racial Equality, *Racial Discrimination in Liverpool City Council: A Report of a Formal Investigation into the Housing Department* (London: CRE, 1989).
73. A. Simpson, *Stacking the Decks: A Study of Race, Inequality and Council Housing in Nottingham* (Nottingham: Nottingham Community Relations Council, 1981); N. Ginsburg, 'Racism and Housing: Concepts and Reality', in P. Braham, A. Rattansi and R. Skellington (eds), in *Racism and Anti-Racism, Inequalities, Opportunities and Policies* (London: Sage, 1992).
74. Commission for Racial Equality, *Living in Terror: A Report of Racial Violence and Harrassment in Housing* (London: CRE, 1987). J. Henderson and V. Karn, *Race, Class and State Housing* (Basingstoke: Macmillan, 1987). D. Phillips, *What Price Equality? A Report on the Allocation of GLC Housing in Tower Hamlets* (London: Greater London Council, 1986).
75. Henderson and Karn, *Race, Class and State Housing*.
76. Commission for Racial Equality, *Racial Discrimination in an Oldham Estate Agency* (London: CRE, 1990).
77. Commission for Racial Equality, *Race and Mortgage Lending: Report of a Formal Investigation* (London: CRE, 1985).
78. Ginsburg, 'Racism and Housing'.
79. Commission for Racial Equality, *Race and Council Housing in Hackney*.
80. Race Relations Act Section 17; Sex Discrimination Act Section 22.
81. Race Relations Act Sections 18 and 19; Sex Discrimination Act Sections 23 and 25.
82. Race Relations Act s. 1.2: 'for the purposes of this Act, segregating a person from other persons on racial grounds is treating him less favourably than they are treated.'
83. Race Relations Act Section 35.

84. Commission for Racial Equality, *Second Review of the Race Relations Act*, pp. 33–4.
85. Commission for Racial Equality, *Second Review of the Race Relations Act*, p. 17.
86. Sex Discrimination Act Section 51.
87. Race Relations Act Section 41.
88. *R v. Entry Clearance Officer* 1983 ex parte Amin 2 All ER 864 HL.
89. Commission for Racial Equality, *Second Review of the Race Relations Act* p. 30.
90. Ibid.
91. Council Directive 75/117 Approximation of laws relating to equal pay for men and women; Council Directive 76/207 On the implementation of the principle of equal treatment for women and men as regards access to employment, vocational training and promotion, and working conditions; Council Directive 79/7 On the Progressive implementation of equal treatment for men and women in matters of social security.
92. Gregory, *Sex, Race and the Law* p. 161.
93. Council Directive 1975/11, Approximation of laws relating to equal pay for men and women.
94. Equal Pay (Amendment) Regulations 1983.
95. 'Equal Pay for Women is Curbed by Ministers', *Independent*, 11 October 1993.
96. Katherine O'Donovan and Erika Szyszczak, *Equality and Sex Discrimination Law* (Oxford: Blackwell, 1988) p. 198.
97. *Dekker* v. *Stiching Vormingcentrum voor Jong Volwassenen Plus* 1990 415 IRLIB 11.
98. *Independent*, 21 January, 1991.
99. *Webb* v. *EMO Air Cargo (UK) Ltd* 1992. Directives which have either not been implemented or have not been properly implemented can be enforced against the state by public sector employees provided they are clear and confer rights upon individuals. Referring to the House of Lords decision in *Duke* v. *GEC Reliance Ltd* (1988 IRLR 118) the Court held that, in relation to a piece of legislation which was not specifically introduced to implement an EC Directive, a British court should not feel constrained to 'distort' domestic legislation to give effect to an EC Directive.
100. O'Donovan and Szyszczak, *Equality and Sex Discrimination Law* p. 204.
101. *R.* v. *Secretary of State for Employment* ex parte EOC, 1994.

Chapter 7: Restructuring British disability laws

1. Civil Rights (Disabled Persons) Bill 1993, Section 1(1).
2. Commission for Racial Equality, *Second Review of the Race Relations Act* (London: CRE, 1992).

3. Ibid. p. 50.
4. E. Topliss and B. Gould, *A Charter for the Disabled* (Oxford: Blackwell & Robertson, 1981) p. 129.
5. Ibid. p. 128.
6. Committee on the Restrictions against Disabled People, *Report by the Committee on the Restrictions Against Disabled People* (Southampton: HMSO, 1982) pp. 16–17 (CORAD Report).
7. C. Barnes, *Disabled People in Britain and Discrimination: A Case for Anti-Discrimination Legislation* (London: Hurst,1991) p. 189.
8. CORAD Report p. 12.
9. HMSO, *A Guide to Fire Regulations in Existing Places of Entertainment and Like Premises* (London: HMSO, 1990) p. 20.
10. British Standards Institute, *British Standards 5588, Part 8: Means of Escape for Disabled People* (London: British Standards Institute 1988).
11. Department of the Environment Circular 74/74 (London: DOE, 1974).
12. A. Rowe (ed.), *Lifetime Homes: Flexible Housing for Successive Generations* (London: Helen Hamlyn Foundation, 1990).
13. Barnes, *Disabled People in Britain* p. 158.
14. Local Government and Housing Act 1989 Section 114.
15. Jill Clarkson, *The Disabled Facilities Grant: Necessary and Appropriate? Reasonable and Practicable?* (London: RADAR, 1992).
16. M. Hirst, *Young People with Disabilities and Their Families* (York: York University Social Policy Unit, 1982); A. Thomas, M. Bax and D. Smythe, *The Health and Social Needs of Young Adults with Physical Disabilities* (Oxford: Blackwell Scientific Publications, 1989).
17. Barnes, *Disabled People in Britain* p. 154.
18. I. Bynoe, M. Oliver and C. Barnes, *Equal Rights for Disabled People – The Case for a New Law* (London: Institute for Public Policy Research, 1991) p. 26.
19. Re Dr Barnardo's Home National Incorporated Association's Application [1955] 7 P&CR 176.
20. Bynoe et al., *Equal Rights for Disabled People* p. 26.
21. Reported in *Community Care*, January 1993.
22. J. Morris, *Freedom to Lose: Housing Policy and People with Disabilities* (London: Shelter, 1988).
23. Jenny Morris, 'No Place to Live', *New Society*, 27 May 1988.
24. L. Laurie, *Conference Report: Building our Lives: Housing, Independent Living and Disabled People* (London: Shelter, 1991) pp. 12–13.
25. Ibid.
26. Ibid.
27. Ibid.
28. Housing Act 1985 Section 59(1).

29. *R* v. *Tower Hamlets LBC* ex parte Begum, House of Lords, *Independent*, 19 March 1993.

30. *Conference Report*, Shelter, p. 9.

31. G. Fulcher, *Disabling Policies? A Comparative Approach to Education Policy and Disability* (London: Falmer, 1989); M. Oliver, 'The Social and Political Context of Educational Policy: The Case of Special Needs' in L. Barton (ed.) *The Politics of Special Educational Needs* (London: Falmer, 1988).

32. M. Warnock, *Special Educational Needs: Report of the Committee of Enquiry into the Education of Children and Young People* (London, HMSO, 1978) p. 37.

33. Fulcher, *Disabling Policies*? p. 164.

34. Education Act 1981 Section 1.

35. Ibid. Section 5.

36. Some children who are recognised as having SEN and requiring additional assistance will not require a formal statement.

37. Fulcher, *Disabling Policies* p. 168.

38. CORAD Report pp. 26–7.

39. Education Act 1993 Sections 177 and 181; Department for Education, *Code of Practice on the Identification and Assessment of Special Educational Needs* (London: DFE, 1994).

40. Quoted in *Times Educational Supplement* 25 May 1978.

41. Education Act 1981 Section 2.

42. Department of Education and Science, *Educational Statistics: Schools* (London: DES, 1990).

43. The figures for disabled children living in institutions were worse, with only 27 per cent receiving integrated schooling. H. Meltzer, M. Smyth and N. Robus, *Disabled Children: Services, Transport and Education* (London: Office of Population and Census Surveys, 1989).

44. Coopers and Lybrand, *Within Reach: Access for Disabled Children to Mainstream Education* (London: Centurion, 1992).

45. Coopers and Lybrand, *Within Reach: The Schools Survey* (London: Centurion, 1993).

46. Ibid. p. 28.

47. Barnes, *Disabled People in Britain* p. 52.

48. Robin Beste, 'Integration Now?', *One in Five*, spring 1992 p. 1.

49. G. Hill, 'If We Really Care', *One in Five*, spring 1992 p. 7.

50. CORAD Report p. 42.

51. B. Goacher, J. Evans, J. Welton, K. Wedell and D. Glaser, *The 1981 Education Act: Policy and Provision for Special Educational Needs: A Report to the Department of Education and Science* (London: University of London Institute of Education, 1986) pp. 22–3.

52. A. Smith, *Opportunities for Students with Disabilities* (London: Public Information Unit, Labour Party, 1990).

53. R. Stowell, *Catching up: A Survey of Provision for Students with Special Educational Needs in Further and Higher Education* (London: SKILL, 1987).
54. Berkeley Planning Associates, *A Study of Accommodations Provided to Handicapped Employees by Federal Contractors* (Berkeley, Calif.: Berkeley Planning Assocs, 1982).
55. Disabled Persons (Employment) Act 1944 Section 9.1.
56. Ibid. Section 9.5.
57. Ibid. Section 1.
58. *Harper* v. *National Coal Board* 1980 IRLR 260.
59. *Griffiths* v. *Hunter* (COIT 1178/166).
60. *Hobson* v. *GEC Telecommunications Ltd* 1985 ICR 777.
61. *Kerr* v. *Atkinson Vehicles (Scotland) Ltd.* 1974 IRLR 361.
62. *Saunders* v. *Omega Lampwork* COIT 1128/23.
63. *Carricks (Caterers) Ltd* v. *Nolan* 1980 IRLR 259.
64. P. Prescott Clarke, *Employment and Handicap* (London: Social and Community Planning Research, 1990). 11 per cent were dismissed, 10 per cent were advised to leave by a doctor, 13 per cent decided for themselves to leave, the remainder left for reasons unrelated to their disability.
65. V. Scott, *Lessons from America* (London: Royal Association for Disability and Rehabilitation, 1994).
66. S. Newman, *Workmates: A Study of Employment Opportunities for Disabled People* (Bishop's Stortford: Mainstream, 1990).
67. Jennifer Hurstfield, *Part-timers under Pressure: Paying the Price of Flexibility* (London: Low Pay Unit, 1987).
68. N. Davoud *Part-time Employment: Time for Recognition, Organisation and Legal Reform* (London: Multiple Sclerosis Society 1980).
69. *Hansard* 27 October 1992, col. 71.
70. A. Hadjipateras and M. Howard, *Too Little, Too Late* (London: Disability Alliance/RADAR, 1992) p. 17.
71. Royal Association for Disability and Rehabilitation, *The Way Ahead: Benefits for Disabled People* (London: RADAR) 1990.
72. A further key problem which the design of DWA acknowledged but failed to solve was the need to provide security by allowing a return to previous benefits if a job fails. Many people who have become disabled or have been out of work for a long time because of their disabilities are uncertain about their capacity to work. The DWA 'linking rule' was supposed to protect the rights of people coming off long-term benefits like Invalidity Benefit or Severe Disablement Allowance by waiving the six-month qualifying period which would normally apply, provided that a claimant was coming off DWA within two years of getting it.
73. Susan Lonsdale, *Invalidity Benefit: An International Comparison* (London: Department of Social Security, 1993).

74. R. Berthoud, *Invalidity Benefit: Where Will the Changes Come From?* (London: Policy Studies Institute, 1993).

75. Ibid. p. 6.

76. Susan Lonsdale, Carli Dessof and Gillian Ferris, *Invalidity Benefit: A Survey of Recipients* (London: Department of Social Security, 1993).

77. Chris Phillipson, *Capitalism and the Construction of Old Age* (London: Macmillan, 1982).

78. Disability Alliance, *A Way out of Poverty and Disability: Moving Towards a Comprehensive Disability Income Scheme* (London: Disability Alliance, 1991) p. 4.

79. P. Thompson, M. Lavery and J. Curtice, *Short Changed by Disability* (London: Disablement Income Group, 1990).

80. Disabled Persons (Services) (No. 2) Bill 1993.

81. See for example M. Oliver and G. Zarb, *Greenwich Personal Assistance Schemes: An Evaluation* (London: University of Greenwich, 1992).

82. Chronically Sick and Disabled Persons Act 1970 Section 1.

83. W. Warburton, *Developing Services for Disabled People* (London: Department of Health, 1990) p. 3.

84. Education of Children Act 1980 Section 8 and accompanying Education School Information Regulations 1981.

85. Department of Education and Science, Circular 1/83 (London: DES, 1983).

86. R. Rogers, *Caught in the Act* (London: Centre for Studies on Integration in Education and The Spastics Society, 1986).

87. Meltzer et al. *Disabled Children.*

88. 'Charities Demand Access to Courts', *Disability Now*, February 1994.

89. Warburton, *Developing Services for Disabled People.*

90. Scott, *Lessons from America* p. 32.

Chapter 8: The prospects for disability rights in Britain

1. R. Scotch, 'Disability Politics and Disability Rights: A Perspective from Great Britain' (unpublished Fellowship Report for the World Rehabilitation Fund, 1986) p. xx.

2. I. Bynoe, M. Oliver and C. Barnes, *Equal Rights for Disabled People – The Case for a New Law* (London: Institute for Public Policy Research, 1991) p. 12.

3. Agnes Fletcher, 'Fighting for the Right to be Different', *New Statesman*, 29 October 1993.

4. 'Special Needs Boy to get Delay Pay Out', *Guardian*, 10 May 1993.

5. '£2000 for Man in Five Year Wait for Aid', *Guardian*, 10 May 1993.

6. 'A Suitable Case for Placement', *Disability Now*, February 1993.

7. Ty Goddard, 'If You Don't Act, Who Will?', *Disability Now*, February 1993.
8. Silver Jubilee Access Committee, *Can Disabled People Go Where You Go?* (London: SJAC, 1979).
9. Committee on Restrictions against Disabled People, *Report by the Committee on Restrictions against Disabled People* (Southampton: HMSO, 1982) (CORAD Report).
10. Bynoe et al., *Equal Rights for Disabled People* p. 57.
11. C. Barnes, *Disabled People in Britain and Discrimination: A Case for Anti-Discrimination Legislation* (London: Hurst, 1991); Bynoe et al., *Equal Rights for Disabled People*.
12. The procedural rules for Private Members Bills make them vulnerable to such tactics, since only a very limited time for debate is allowed, and if it overruns the Bill fails.
13. *Hansard*, 26 February 1993 col. 1179.
14. Ibid. col. 1177.
15. *Hansard*, 6 May 1994 col. 1004.
16. Department of Employment, *Employment and Training for People with Disabilities* (London: DoE,1990).
17. Employment Committee, House of Commons, First Report: *Disability and Employment* (House of Commons Paper 35, 1990).
18. The Law Society's Employment Law Committee, *Disability Discrimination and Employment Law* (London: Law Society, 1992).
19. Ibid. p. 16.
20. Employers Forum on Disability (EFD), *The Need for Partnership* (London: EFD, 1993)
21. Employers Forum on Disability, 'Employers Call for Fresh Partnership with Government and Disabled People', press release, 6 December 1993.
22. A. Fletcher, 'Fighting for the Right to be Different', *New Statesman*, 29 October 1993.
23. *Sun*, 17 February 1993.
24. Commission of the European Communities, 'The Community Charter of Fundamental Social Rights for Workers', Brussels, 1989.
25. Council Recommendation 86/379/EEC OJ.
26. Commission of the European Communities Com. (88) 746 Final, 15 December 1988.
27. Conclusions of the Council of Ministers on the Employment of Disabled People in the Community, OJ C173/1–2, 8 July 1989.
28. Ibid.
29. Ibid.
30. N. Lunt and P. Thornton, *Employment Policies for Disabled People: A Review of Legislation and Services in Fifteen Countries* (Employment Department Research Series No. 16) (York: Social Policy Research Unit, University of York, 1993).

31. Ibid. p. 179.
32. *US News & World Reports*, 18 September 1989.
33. Evan Kemp, Speech to Employers' Banquet of the President's Committee on the Employment of the Handicapped, 5 May 1988.
34. Frank Bowe, Employment Climate' (unpublished Report, 1988).
35. J. Martin, A. White and H. Meltzer, *Disabled Adults: Services, Transport and Employment* (London: Office of Population Censuses and Surveys, 1989).
36. Labour Force Survey, March 1993.
37. Kemp, Speech to President's Committee.
38. Bowe, 'Employment Climate'.
39. Barnes, *Disabled People in Britain* p. 224.
40. Scott, *Lessons from America* (London: Royal Association for Disability and Rehabilitation, 1994) pp. 31–2.
41. Tom Shakespear of REGARD, quoted in Fletcher, 'Fighting for the Right to be Different'.
42. See Chapter 2.

Bibliography

Access Committee for England *Building Homes for Successive Generations* (London: Access Committee for England, 1992)

Adams, A. *Towards Fair Employment and the EEOC: A study of Compliance Procedures under Title VII of the Civil Rights Act 1965* (Washington: EEOC, 1972)

Adkins, G. and Pati, J. 'Hire the Handicapped – Compliance is Good Business', *Harvard Business Review*, January 1980

Barnes, Colin, *Disabled People in Britain and Discrimination: A Case for Anti-Discrimination Legislation* (London: Hurst, 1991)

Barnes, Colin, *Disabling Imagery and the Media: An Exploration of the Principles for Media Representations of Disabled People* (London: BCODP, 1992)

Barton, L. (ed.) *The Politics of Special Educational Needs* (London: Falmer, 1988)

Barton, L. and Tomlinson, S. (eds) *Special Education: Policy, Practices and Social Issues* (London: Harper & Row, 1981)

Berkeley Planning Associates *A Study of Accommodations Provided to Handicapped Employees* (Berkeley: Berkeley Planning Assocs, 1982)

Berkowitz, M. and Hill, A. *Disability in the Labor Market* (New York: Praeger, 1986)

Berthoud, R. *Invalidity Benefit: Where will the Changes Come From?* (London: Policy Studies Institute, 1993)

Beste, R. 'Integration Now?', *One in Five*, Spring 1992

Bindman, G. 'Appointing Judges without Discrimination', *New Law Journal*, 13 December 1991

Blumenrosen, A. 'Towards Effective Administration of New Regulatory Statutes', *Administrative Law Review* 2 (1977)

Blumenrosen, A. 'The Legacy of Griggs: Social Progress and Subjective Judgment', *Chicago–Kent Law Review* 82 (1986)

Bowe, F. *Handicapping America* (New York: Harper & Row, 1978)

Bowe, F. *Civil Rights Issues for Handicapped Americans* (New York: Harper & Row, 1980)

Bowe, F. 'Employment Climate' (unpublished Report, 1988)

Bradfield, J. 'Undue Hardship: Title 1 ADA', *Fordham Law Review* 1 (1990)

Braham, P., Rattansi, A. and Skellington, R. (eds) *Racism and Anti-Racism, Inequalities, Opportunities and Policies* (London: Sage, 1992)

British Standards Institute, *British Standards 5588, Part 8: Means of Escape for Disabled People* (London: British Standards Institute, 1988)

Brodin, J. 'Cost, Profit and the Equal Opportunity', *Notre Dame Law Review* 62 (1987)

Brown, C. and Gay, P. *Racial Discrimination: 17 Years after the Act* (London: Policy Studies Institute, 1986)

Brown, H. and Smith, H. 'Whose Life is it Anyway? Community Care Policy', *Disability, Handicap and Society* (1989)

Burgdorf, R. and Bell, C. *Accommodating the Spectrum of Abilities* (Washington, DC: US Commission for Civil Rights, 1983)

Burstein, P. and Monaghan, K. 'Equal Opportunity and the Mobilization of Law', *Law and Society Review*, 20 (1986)

Business Week, 28 October 1991

Bynoe, I., Oliver, M. and Barnes, C. *Equal Rights for Disabled People – The Case for a New Law* (London: Institute for Public Policy Research, 1991)

Chambers, G. and Horton, C. *Promoting Sex Equality: The Role of Industrial Tribunals* (London: Policy Studies Institute, 1990)

Clarkson, J. *The Disabled Facilities Grant: Necessary and Appropriate? Reasonable and Practicable?* (London: RADAR, 1992)

Commission for Racial Equality *Race and Council Housing in Hackney: Report of a Formal Investigation* (London: CRE, 1984)

Commission for Racial Equality *The Race Relations Code of Practice in Employment* (London: CRE, 1984)

Commission for Racial Equality *Race and Mortgage Lending: Report of a Formal Investigation* (London: CRE, 1985)

Commission for Racial Equality *Race and Housing in Liverpool*, 2nd edn. (London: CRE, 1986)

Commission for Racial Equality *Living in Terror: A Report of racial Violence and Harrassment in Housing* (London: CRE, 1987)

Commission for Racial Equality *Racial Discrimination in Liverpool City Council: A Report of a Formal Investigation into the Housing Department* (London: CRE, 1989)

Commission for Racial Equality *Racial Discrimination in an Oldham Estate Agency* (London: CRE, 1990)

Commission for Racial Equality *Second Review of the Race Relations Act 1976: A Consultative Paper* (London: CRE, 1991)

Commission for Racial Equality *Second Review of the Race Relations Act* (London: CRE, 1992)

Commission for Racial Equality *Race through the 90s* (London: CRE, 1993)

Commission of the European Communities Com (88) 746 Final (Luxembourg: Commission of the EC, 15 December 1988)

Commission of the European Communities 'The Community Charter of Fundamental Social Rights for Workers', (Brussels, 1989)

Committee on Restrictions Against Disabled People *Report by the Committee on Restrictions Against Disabled People* (Southampton: HMSO, 1982)

Compton, R. and Sanderson, K. *Gendered Jobs and Social Change* (London: Unwin Hyman, 1990)

Conaghan, J. and Mansell, W. 'Tort Law' in Grigg-Spall, I. and Ireland, P. (eds), *The Critical Lawyers Handbook* (London: Pluto Press, 1992)

Conference of Indian Organizations *Double Bind: To be Disabled and Asian* (London: Conference of Indian Organizations, 1987)

Congressional Quarterly Researcher 'The Disabilities Act', 1, (32), 27 December 1991

Cooper, J. *Key Guide to Information Sources in Public Law* (London: Mansell, 1991)

Cooper, J. and Dhavan, R. *Public Interest Law* (Oxford: Blackwell, 1986)

Coopers and Lybrand *Within Reach: Access for Disabled Children to Mainstream Education* (London: Centurion, 1992)

Coopers and Lybrand *Within Reach: The Schools Survey* (London: Centurion, 1993)

Cotterell, R. *The Sociology of Law: An Introduction* 2nd edn. (London: Butterworths, 1992)

Council of Ministers of the European Community *Recommendation on the Employment of Disabled People in the Community* (OJ L225/43 of 12 August 1986)

Council of Ministers of the European Community *Conclusions of the Council on the Employment of Disabled People in the Community* (OJ C 173/1 of 8 July 1989)

Crowther, M. *The Workhouse System 1834–1929: The History of an English Institution* (London: Methuen, 1983)

Curran, B. *The Legal Needs of the Public* (Chicago: American Bar Foundation, 1977)

Dahl, R. *Dilemmas of Pluralist Democracy: Autonomy and Control* (New Haven, Mass.: Yale University Press, 1982)

Davoud, N. *Part-time Employment: Time for Recognition, Organisation and Legal Reform* (London: Multiple Sclerosis Society, 1980)

De Tocqueville, A. *Democracy in America*, ed. Phillip Bradley (New York: Knopf, 1945)

Department of Education and Science *Educational Statistics: Schools* (London: DES, 1990)

Department for Education *Code of Practice on the Identification and Assessment of Special Educational Needs* (London: DFE, 1994)

Department of Employment, *Employment and Training for People with Disabilities* (London: DoE, 1990)

Department of the Environment Circular 74/74 (London: Department of the Environment 1974)

Dickens, L. *Whose Flexibility? Discrimination and Equality Issues in Atypical Work* (London: Institute of Employment Rights, 1992)

Disability Alliance *A Way out of Poverty and Disability: Moving towards a Comprehensive Disability Income Scheme* (London: Disability Alliance, 1991)

Disability Now 'Charities Demand Access to Courts', February 1994

Disabled Persons Transport Advisory Committee *Making Buses More Suitable for Elderly and Ambulant Disabled People* (London: DPTAC, 1988)

Disabled Persons Transport Advisory Committee *Public Transport and the Missing Six Millions: What Can be Learned?* (London: DPTAC, 1989)

Doyal, L. with Pennell, I. *The Political Economy of Health* (London: Pluto Press, 1979)

Drummond, M. 'Positive Discrimination', *Guardian,* 1 March 1994

Eastwood, M. 'The Double Standard of Justice: Women's Rights under the Constitution', *Valparaiso University Law Review* 5(2) (1971)

Edgerton, R. *Deviance: A Cross-Cultural Perspective* (London: Benjamin, 1976)

Eichner, M. 'Getting Women Work which isn't Women's Work: Challenging Biases in the Workplace', *Yale Law Journal* 97 (1988)

Eisenberg, T. 'Integration Models and Trial Outcomes in Civil Rights and Prisoner Cases', *Georgetown Law Review* 77 (1989)

Employment Department, *Labour Force Survey,* March 1993

Employers Forum on Disability *The Need for Partnership* (London: EFD, 1993)

Employers Forum on Disability 'Employers Call for Fresh Partnership with Government and Disabled People', press release, 6 December 1993

Employment Committee, House of Commons, *First Report: Disability and Employment* (House of Commons Paper 35, 1990)

Employment Gazette, 'Ethnic Origins and the Labour Market', March 1990

Equal Employment Opportunity Commission 'EEOC marks first year of enforcing the ADA in the Workplace', Washington, DC, press release, 23 July 1993

Equal Opportunities Commission *Women and Men in Britain: A Statistical Profile* (Manchester: EOC, 1986)

Equal Opportunities Commission *Equal Treatment for Men and Women: Strengthening the Acts: Formal Proposals* (Manchester: EOC, 1988)

Equal Opportunities Commission *Annual Report 1992: The Equality Challenge* (Manchester: EOC, 1992)

Equal Opportunities Review, 'Compensation Awards: Employers Pay More for Race and Sex Bias', No. 49, May/June 1993

Equal Opportunities Review, 'Maternity Proposals Will Increase Sex Bias', No. 52 November/December 1993

Farber, B. *Mental Handicap: Its Social Context and Social Consequences* (Boston, Mass: Houghton Mifflin, 1986)

Finley, L. 'Transcending Equality Theory: A Way out of the Maternity and Workplace Debate', *Colorado Law Review* 86 (1986)

Finklestein, V. *Attitudes and Disabled People: Issues for Discussion* (New York: World Rehabilitation Fund, 1980)

Fitzpatrick, P. 'Racism and the Innocence of Law', in Fitzpatrick, P. and Hunt, A. (eds), *Critical Legal Studies* (Oxford: Blackwell, 1987)

Fletcher, A. 'Fighting For the Right to be Different', *New Statesman,* 29 October 1993

Foner, E. *A Short History of Reconstruction* (New York: Harper & Row, 1990)

Foucault, M. *Madness and Civilisation: A History of Insanity in the Age of Reason* (London: Tavistock, 1967)

Foucault, M. *Archeology of Knowledge* (New York: Pantheon, 1972)

Foucault M. *Power/Knowledge: Selected Interviews and Other Writings 1972–77* (Brighton: Wheatsheaf, 1980)

Fuchs, V. *Women's Quest for Equality* (Cambridge, Mass.: Harvard University Press, 1980)

Fulcher, G. *Disabling Policies? A Comparative Approach to Education Policy and Disability* (London: Falmer, 1989)

Gallup Organization, *Baseline Study to Determine Businesses' Attitudes, Awareness and Reaction to the Americans with Disabilities Act* (Princeton, NJ: Gallup, 1992)

Gardner, J. *No Offence?* (London: Industrial Society, 1993)

Gartner A. and Joe, T. *Images of the Disabled: Disabling Images* (New York: Praeger, 1987)

Genn, H. and Genn, Y. *The Effectiveness of Representation at Tribunals: Report to the Lord Chancellor* (London: Lord Chancellor's Department, 1989)

Gerse, S. 'Mending the Rehabilitation Act of 1973', *University of Illinois Law Review* (1982)

Gibbons, J. 'Residential Care for Mentally Ill Adults', in Sinclair, I. (ed.), *Residential Care: The Research Reviewed,* Literature surveys commissioned by the Independent Review of Residential Care (London: National Institute for Social Work/HMSO, 1988)

Gilligan, C. *In a Different Voice* (London: Harvard University Press, 1982)

Ginsburg, N. 'Racism and Housing: Concepts and Reality', in Braham, P., Rattansi, A. and Skellington, R. (eds) *Racism and Anti-Racism, Inequalities, Opportunities and Policies* (London: Sage, 1992)

Gittler, A. 'Fair Employment and the Handicapped: A Legal Perspective', *De Paul Law Review* 27 (1978)

Goacher B., Evans, J., Welton, J., Wedell, K. and Glaser, D. *The 1981 Education Act: Policy and Provision for Special Educational Needs: A Report to the Department of Education and Science* (London: University of London Institute of Education, 1986)

Goddard, T. 'If You Don't Act, Who Will?', *Disability Now*, February 1993

Gostin L. (ed.) *Civil Liberties in Conflict* (London: Routledge, 1988)

Gough, I. *The Political Economy of the Welfare State* (London: Macmillan, 1981)

Gregory, J. *Sex, Race and the Law: Legislating for Equality* (London: Sage, 1987)

Gregory, J. *Trial by Ordeal: A Study of People who Lose Equal Pay and Sex Discrimination Cases in the Industrial Tribunals during 1985 and 1986* (London: HMSO, 1989)

Griffith, J. A.G. *The Politics of the Judiciary*, 2nd edn. (London: Fontana, 1981)

Grigg-Spall, I. and Ireland P. (eds) *The Critical Lawyers Handbook* (London: Pluto Press, 1992)

Guardian, 'Special Needs Boy to Get Delay Pay Out', 10 May 1993

Guardian, 'A Suitable Case for Placement', 6 July 1993

Guardian, 'Appointing Judges Without Discrimination', 1 March 1994

Hadjipateras, A. and Howard, M. *Too Little, Too Late* (London: Disability Alliance/RADAR, 1992)

Hahn, H. *Issues of Equality: European Perceptions of Employment Policy and Disabled Persons* (New York: World Rehabilitation Fund, 1984)

Hanks, J. and Hanks, L. 'The Physically Handicapped in Certain Non-Occidental Societies', in Philips, W. and Rosenberg, J. (eds) *Social Scientists and the Physically Handicapped* (London: Arno Press, 1980)

Hansard, 27 October 1992

Hansard, 26 February 1993

Harlow, C. and Rawlings, R. *Pressure through Law* (London: Routledge, 1992)

Harris, L. and Associates *Disabled Americans' Self-perceptions: Bringing Disabled Americans into the Mainstream* (New York: Harris, 1986)

Harrison, F. *The Young Disabled Adult: The Use of Residential Homes and Hospital Units for the Age Group 16–64: A Report for the Royal College of Physicians* (London: Royal College of Physicians, 1986)

Harvard Law Review Note: 'Employment Discrimination against the Handicapped: An Essay in Legal Evasiveness' 97 (1984)

Hearn, K. 'Disabled Lesbians are Here to Stay' in Kaufman, T. and Lincoln, P. (eds) *High Risk Lives* (Bridport: Prism Press, 1991)

Henderson, J. and Karn, V. *Race, Class and State Housing* (Basingstoke: Macmillan, 1987)

Hill, G. 'If We Really Care', *One in Five*, Spring 1992

Hippololitus, P. *College Bound Freshmen with Disabilities Preparing for Employment: A Statistical Profile* (Washington, DC: President's Committee on the Employment of the Handicapped and the American Council for Education, 1985)

Hirst, M. *Young People with Disabilities and their Families* (York: York University Social Policy Unit, 1982)

HMSO, *A Guide to Fire Regulations in Existing Places of Entertainment and Like Premises* (London: HMSO 1990)

Holland, K. *Judicial Activism in Comparative Perspective* (London: Macmillan, 1991)

Honey, S., Meager, N. and Williams, M. *Employers' Attitudes towards People with Disabilities* (Brighton: Institute of Manpower Studies, University of Sussex 1993)

House of Commons Standing Advisory Committee on Human Rights, *Religious and Political Discrimination and Equal Opportunity in Northern Ireland* Cm. 237 (London: HMSO, 1987)

Howards, I., Brahm, J. and Naagi, S. *Disability from Social Program to Federal Program* (New York: Praeger, 1980)

Hurstfield, J. *Part-timers under Pressure: Paying the Price of Flexibility* (London: Low Pay Unit, 1987)

Illich, I. *Medical Nemesis: The Expropriation of Health* (London: Calder & Boyars, 1975)

Independent, 10 September 1993

Independent, 'Equal Pay for Women is Curbed by Ministers', 11 October 1993

Institute of Personnel Management, *Contract Compliance – The UK Experience* (London: Income Data Services, 1987)

Johnson, M. 'The Rehabilitation Act and Disabled Workers', in Berkowitz, M. and Hill, A. (eds) *Disability in the Labor Market* (New York: Praeger, 1986)

Johnson, M. 'Enabling Act: Americans with Disabilities Act', *The Nation*, 28 November 1989

Katzman, R. *Institutional Disability: The Saga of Transportation Policy for the Disabled* (Washington, DC: Brookings Institute, 1986)

Kennedy, D. 'Legal Education as Training for Hierarchy', in Grigg-Spall, I. and Ireland, P. (eds) *The Critical Lawyers Handbook* (London: Pluto Press, 1992)

Kent, D. 'In Search of a Heroine: Images of Women with Disabilities in Fiction and Drama' in Asch, A. and Fine, M. (eds) *Women with Disabilities: Essays in Psychology, Culture and Politics* (Philadelphia: Temple University Press, 1988)

Kettle, M. *Survey of the Association of Disabled Professionals* (Surrey: Association of Disabled Professionals, 1975)

Kettle, M. *Disabled People and their Employment: A Review of Research into the Performance of Disabled People at Work* (Surrey: Association of Disabled Professionals, 1979)

Krieger, L. and Cooney, P. 'The Miller Wohl Controversy: Equal Treatment, Positive Action and the Meaning of Women's Equality, *Golden Gate University Law Review* 13 (513) (1983)

Kumar, V. *Industrial Tribunal Applicants under the Race Relations Act 1976* (London: CRE, 1986)

Laurie, L. Conference Report: *Building Our Lives: Housing, Independent Living and Disabled People* (London: Shelter, 1991)

Law Society's Employment Law Committee *Disability Discrimination and Employment Law* (London: Law Society, 1992)

Law Society Solicitors with Disabilities Group, 'Survey', *Educare*, November 1992

Lawrence, L. 'The Id, Ego and Equal Protection: Reckoning with Unconscious Racism', *Stanford Law Review* 39 (1987)

Leonard, A. *Judging Inequality: The Effectiveness of the Tribunal System in Sex Discrimination and Equal Pay Cases* (London: Cobden Trust, 1987)

Lester, A. *A British Bill of Rights* (London: Institute of Public Policy Research, 1990)

Lester, A. and Bindman, G. *Race and the Law* (Harmondsworth: Penguin, 1972)

Liggett, H. 'The Efficacy of State Fair Employment Commissions', *Industrial and Labour Relations Research*, 22 (1968–9)

Liggett, H. 'Stars are Not Born: An Interactive Approach to the Politics of Disability', *Disability, Handicap and Society*, 3, 3 (1988)

Lonsdale, S. *Women and Disability* (London: Macmillan, 1990)

Lonsdale, S. *Invalidity Benefit: An International Comparison* (London: Department of Social Security, 1993)

Lonsdale, S., Dessof, C. and Ferris, G. *Invalidity Benefit: A Survey of Recipients* (London: Department of Social Security, 1993)

Lord Chancellor's Department, *Judicial Appointments – The Lord Chancellor's Policies and Procedures* (London: Lord Chancellor's Department, 1990)

Lunt, N. and Thornton, P. *Employment Policies for Disabled People: A Review of Legislation and Services in Fifteen Countries* (Employment Department Research Series No. 16) (York: Social Policy Research Unit, University of York, 1993)

Lustgarten, L. and Edwards, J. 'Racial Equality and the Limits of the Law' in Braham, P., Rattansi, A. and Skellington, R. (eds) *Racism and Anti-Racism: Inequalities, Opportunities and Policies* (London: Sage, 1992)

McCluskey, M. 'Rethinking Equality and Difference: Disability Discrimination in Public Transport', *Yale Law Journal* 97 (1988)

MacKinnon, C. *Feminism Unmodified: Discourses on Life and Law* (Cambridge, Mass.: Harvard University Press, 1987)

McCrudden, C. 'The Northern Ireland Fair Employment White Paper: A Critical Assessment', *Industrial Law Journal* 17 (1988)

McCrudden, C., Smith, D. and Brown, C. *Racial Justice at Work: Enforcement of the Race Relations Act 1976* (London: Policy Studies Institute, 1991)

Marshall, R., Knapp, C. and Glover, R. *Employment Discrimination: The Impact of Legal and Administrative Remedies* (New York: Praeger, 1978)

Martin J., Meltzer, H. and Elliott, D. *The Prevalence of Disability amongst Adults* (London: Office of Population Censuses and Surveys, 1988)

Martin J., White, A. and Meltzer, H. *Disabled Adults: Services, Transport and Employment* (London: Office of Population Censuses and Surveys, 1989)

Martin, M. 'Note: Accommodating the Handicapped: The Meaning of Discrimination under s504 of the Rehabilitation Act', *New York University Law Review* 55 (1980)

Meehan, E. *Women's Rights at Work: Campaigns and Policy in Britain and the United States* (Basingstoke: Macmillan, 1985)

Meltzer, H., Smyth, M. and Robus, N. *Disabled Children: Services, Transport and Education* (London: Office of Population and Census Surveys, 1989)

Morrel, J. *The Employment of People with Disabilities: Research into the Policies and Practices of Employers* (Sheffield: Employment Department, 1990)

Morris, J. 'No place to live', *New Society*, 27 May 1988

Morris, J. *Freedom to Lose: Housing Policy and People with Disabilities* (London: Shelter, 1988)

Morris, J. *Able Lives: Women's Experience of Paralysis* (London: Women's Press, 1989)

Morris, J. *Pride against Prejudice: Transforming Attitudes to Disability* (London: Women's Press, 1991)

National Council on Disability *Towards Independence* (Washington, DC: National Council on Disability, 1986)

National Council on Disability *On the Threshold of Independence* (Washington, DC: National Council on Disability, 1988)

National Council on Disability *ADA Watch – Year One: A Report to the President and Congress on Progress in Implementing the Americans with Disabilities Act* (Washington, DC: National Council on Disability, 1993)

National Review, 11 June 1990

Newman, S. *Workmates: A Study of Employment Opportunities for Disabled People* (Bishop's Stortford: Mainstream, 1990)

O'Donovan, K. and Szyszczak, E. *Equality and Sex Discrimination Law* (Oxford: Blackwell, 1988)

Oliver, M. 'The Social and Political Context of Educational Policy: The Case of Special Needs', in Barton, L. (ed.) *The Politics of Special Educational Needs* (London: Falmer, 1988)

Oliver, M. *The Politics of Disablement* (Basingstoke: Macmillan, 1990)

Oliver, M. 'Cock-up or Conspiracy?' *Therapy Weekly*, 11 March 1993

Oliver, M. and Zarb, G. *Greenwich Personal Assistance Schemes: An Evaluation* (London: University of Greenwich, 1992)

Pashunakis, E. *Law and Marxism: A General Theory* (London: Ink Links, 1987)

Percy, S. Disability, *Civil Rights and Public Policy: The Politics of Implementation* (Montgomery: University of Alabama Press, 1989)

Phillips, D. *What Price Equality? A Report on the Allocation of GLC Housing in Tower Hamlets* (London: Greater London Council, 1986)

Prescott Clarke, P. *Employment and Handicap* (London: Social and Community Planning Research, 1990)

Rasky, A. 'How the Disabled Sold Congress on a Bill of Rights', *New York Times*, 17 September 1989

Rebell, M. 'Structural Discrimination and the Disabled', *Georgetown Law Journal* 74 (1986)

Rogers R. *Caught in the Act* (London: Centre for Studies on Integration in Education and The Spastics Society, 1986)

Rothman, D. *The Discovery of the Asylum* (Boston, Mass.: Little, Brown, 1971)

Rowe A. (ed.), *Lifetime Homes: Flexible Housing for Successive Generations* (London: Helen Hamlyn Foundation, 1990)

Royal Association for Disability and Rehabilitation *The Way Ahead: Benefits for Disabled People* (London: RADAR,1990)

Royal Association in Aid of Deaf People *A Change in Approach: A Report on the Experiences of Deaf People from Black and Ethnic Minorities* (London: RAD, 1991)

Ryan, J. and Thomas, F. *The Politics of Mental Handicap* (Harmondsworth: Penguin, 1980)

Sage, Adam 'Black Barristers Face Exam Bias', *Independent*, 10 September 1993.

Saxton, M. and Howe, F. (eds) *With Wings* (London: Virago, 1988)

Scales, A. 'The Emergence of Feminist Jurisprudence', *Yale Law Journal* 95 (1986)

Schneider, E. 'The Dialectics of Rights and Politics: Perspectives from the Women's Movement', *New York Univ. Law Review* 61 (1986)

Scotch, R. *From Goodwill to Civil Rights: Transforming Federal Disability Policy* (Philadelphia: Temple University Press, 1984)

Scotch, R. 'Disability Politics and Disability Rights: A Perspective from Great Britain' (Unpublished Fellowship Report for the World Rehabilitation Fund, 1986)

Scott, R. *The Making of Blind Men: A Study of Adult Socialization* (New York: Russell Sage Foundation, 1969)

Scott, V. *Lessons from America* (London: Royal Association for Disability and Rehabilitation, 1994)

Sedgwick, P. *Psycho Politics* (London: Pluto Press, 1982)

Silver Jubilee Access Committee, *Can Disabled People Go Where You Go?* (London: SJAC, 1979)

Simpson, A. *Stacking the Decks: A Study of Race, Inequality and Council Housing in Nottingham* (Nottingham: Nottingham Community Relations Council, 1981)

Sinclair, I. (ed.), *Residential Care: The Research Reviewed*, literature surveys commissioned by the Independent Review of Residential Care (London: National Institute for Social Work/HMSO, 1988)

Smart, C. *Feminism and the Power of Law* (London: Routledge, 1989)

Smith, A. *Opportunities for Students with Disabilities* (London: Public Information Unit, Labour Party, 1990)

Spencer, A. and Podmore, D. *In a Man's: World, Essays on Women in Male Dominated Professions* (London: Tavistock, 1987)

Squibb, P. 'A Theoretical Structuralist Approach to Special Education' in Barton, L. and Tomlinson, S. (eds) *Special Education: Policy, Practices and Social Issues* (London: Harper & Row, 1981)

Stone, D. *The Disabled State* (Basingstoke: Macmillan, 1984)

Stowell, R. *Catching Up: A Survey of Provision for Students with Special Educational Needs in Further and Higher Education* (London: SKILL, 1987)

Sun, 17 February 1993

Szaz, T. *The Myth of Mental Illness* (New York: Harper & Row, 1961)

Taub, N. and Williams, W. 'Will Equality Require More than Assimilation, Accommodation or Separation from the Existing Strucure?', *Rutger Law Review* 37 (1987)

Therapy Weekly, 'CSP Pledge on Equality Issues' 20 November 1992

Thomas, A., Bax, M. and Smythe, D. *The Health and Social Needs of Young Adults with Physical Disabilities* (Oxford: Blackwell Scientific Publications, 1989)

Thompson, P., Lavery, M. and Curtice, J. *Short Changed by Disability* (London: Disablement Income Group, 1990)

Thomson, A. 'Foreword: Critical Approaches to Law: Who Needs Legal Theory?', in Grigg-Spall, I. and Ireland, P. (eds) *The Critical Lawyers Handbook* (London: Pluto Press, 1992)

Times Educational Supplement 25 May 1978

Topliss, E. and Gould, B. *A Charter for the Disabled* (Oxford: Blackwell & Robertson, 1981)

Treiman, D. and Hartman, H. *Women, Work and Wages* (Washington, DC: National Academy Press, 1981)

TUC, *Women in the Labour Market* (London: TUC, 1983)

Tucker, B. 'Section 504 of the Rehabilitation after Ten Years of Enforcement: The Past and the Future', *University of Illinois Law Review*, 4 (1989)

Unger, R. *Critical Legal Studies Movement* (Cambridge: Harvard University Press, 1986)

Union of the Physically Impaired against Segregation *Fundamental Principles of Disability* (London: UPIAS, 1976)

US Department of Labor, *The Performance of Physically Impaired Workers in Manufacturing Industries* (Washington, DC: US Department of Labor, 1948)

US Department of Transportation, *Preliminary Cost Analysis, ADA Vehicle Accessibility Requirements* (Washington, DC: DOT, 1990)

US General Accounting Office, *Report to the Subcommittee on Select Education and Civil Rights, Committee on Education and Labor, House of Representatives: Americans with Disabilities Act, Initial Accessibility Good but Important Barriers Remain* (Washington: US General Accounting Office, 1993)

US News & World Reports 18 September 1989

USA Today 22 July 1993

Wagstaff, J. 'Getting Around London', *Contact*, 65 (1990)

Wall Street Journal, 'Employment Act for Lawyers', 11 September 1989

Wallace, P. (ed.) *Equal Employment Opportunity and the AT & T case* (Cambridge, Mass.: MIT Press, 1976)

Warburton, W. *Developing Services for Disabled People* (London: Department of Health, 1990)

Warnock, M. *Special Educational Needs: Report of the Committee of Enquiry into the Education of Children and Young People* (London: HMSO, 1978)

Weeks, J. *Sex, Politics and Society: The Regulation of Sexuality since 1800*, 2nd edn. (London: Longman, 1989)

West, J. *Millbank Quarterly* 69 (1991)

Which?, 'No Go', June 1990

Williams, P. 'Alchemical Notes: Reconstructing Ideals from Deconstructed Rights', *Harvard Civil Rights–Civil Liberties Review* 22 (1987)

Wilson, E. *Only Halfway to Paradise* (London: Tavistock, 1980)

Witz, A. *Professions and Patriarchy* (London: Routledge, 1992)

Yellin, E. 'The Recent History and Immediate Future of Employment amongst People with Disabilities' in J. West, *Millbank Quarterly* 69 (1991)

Index